HOW TO LOSE WEIGHT FAST

Dr. Shikha Singh

Published By

Invincible Publication Pvt. Ltd.

Published by:

Invincible Publication Pvt.Ltd.

201A, SAS Tower, Sector 38, Gurugram, Haryana – 122003

Phone: +91-124-4034247, +91 9599066061

Website : www.invinciblepublishers.com

Sales Office : - 4760-61/23, Basement, Pratap Street, Ansari Road,

Daryaganj, New Delhi - 110002

Phone: +91-11-40198405

Email: invinciblepublishers@gmail.com

ISBN : 978-93-58863-27-7

Book Name : How to Lose Weight Fast

By - Shikha Singh

First Edition: January 2024

About the book

Weight loss is a slippery slope. It's like, four steps forward and three steps back, kind of a deal. With so much advice from our relatives, friends and of course the internet on the ways of losing weight, we often feel confused about one of the most important and fundamental aspects of our life, i.e food. Are you also tired of falling back into the same pit; fat, fit and fat again? Things work for you temporarily but then it goes back to square one? This pattern occurs when we only treat the symptom and not the root cause of obesity. I say, weight loss is a multi-layered process but most often it is only dealt with at the surface. With my expertise as a leading Nutritionist and my five secret golden rules, I am here to make your journey to weight loss fun, easy and permanent. A journey where you will learn to take care of your health and your weight on your own without relying on supplements, crash diets and workouts. This book will help you to meet a healthier, more beautiful and a more aware 'You'. All we need is to go back to basics and maybe even unlearn a few things. But I promise that this knowledge will change your take on weight loss and help you look at it from a solution based approach rooted into the understanding of the cause of your problem. No diets, no overindulging exercises, no boycotting tasty food, just a holistic life with nature and its best medicine, food.

About the author

The author of How to Lose Weight Fast, Shikha Singh is a leading Doctor & a Certified Clinical Nutritionist who has helped thousands of individuals on their journey to weight loss. She stands for science-backed nutrition combined with home cooked food as the best medicine for weight loss and healing oneself from within. Once weighing 110 kilos herself, she understands the struggles that one faces in this journey. This is why her efforts come from a place of compassion and are driven by a mission to help ease the life of people that are weighed down by obesity everyday. Her unique way of using science and traditional knowledge without compromising on the demands of modern lifestyle, is what makes her popular amongst the millions of viewership on her youtube channel.

Disclaimer

Any advice or guideline given through this book is a general advisory to help an individual intending to lose weight. It is essential that the reader implements or enacts the advice and guidelines by being mindful of their medical conditions and after consultation with their health provider. The reader with serious health disorders and other underlying medical conditions should practice caution before adopting any new dietary habits or lifestyle changes. In general readers should also consult and confirm their conclusions drawn from any section of this book with a doctor before finalizing them based on their personal views. Dr. Shikha as a certified clinician has tried her best to bring science based knowledge and solutions to the readers on their weight loss journey. And any other motive is not implied or intended by the content of this book.

TABLE OF CONTENT

Chapter 1 : What is the weight problem?

Chapter 2 : 5 Golden Rules to weight loss

Chapter 3 : What makes a good diet for weight loss?

Chapter 4 : Do you know these additionals of weight loss?

Chapter 5 : Can I lose weight If I have.....?

Chapter 6 : Diet plan for Teenagers

Chapter 7 : A chapter dedicated to my women readers!

Introduction

What do you need to lose weight? A crash diet, days of fasting, boring boiled food, lots of exercise? I say, weight loss doesn't come with these torturous things. Rather it's fun, it's exciting and it is full of tasty yet healthy food. No more starving yourself, no more killing the cravings, I'll teach you how to enjoy this process and not beat yourself to defeat with the half cooked knowledge out there.

Our bodies are excellent mirrors of the states of our internal health. What inputs we put inside in terms of food, supplements, medicines etc., our shape, size, resilience and an overall personality comes out as an output of it. Your food and your lifestyle do not just affect your body, they have a huge impact on your mind as well. You must be familiar with the old saying, 'you are what you eat'.

The issue of obesity is not an isolated event that occurs in one's life. It's not a result of one factor but it has a bigger story to tell. 'Ahaar' your food, 'achar' your habits, 'vichar' your thoughts and 'vihar' your recreation, are four pillars of a healthy lifestyle. An imbalance in these factors, together form the blueprint for the occurrence of obesity in your life. Obesity is not a disease, it's a symptom of things that are going wrong inside. But gradually this symptom itself becomes the cause of problems and diseases.

How many times have you tried a crash diet, or keto, or tried going to the gym and tried this food or that food? And how many times have you found yourself circling back to the same scales on your weighing machine? These are all temporary fixes. Additionally they run a chase on your money, your time and effort.

Someone will tell you to eat one thing but it messes with your system. The other will tell you to eat something else, which will work for you but you remain confused regarding the diet size of that edible. At times a rigorous routine of physical activity is suggested to a body that can only take a brisk walk of 10-20 minutes. There is so much information out there, something works for someone does not guarantee that it will work for you too. It's not a matter of the right thing but a right match. There is no universality when it comes to the choices and the likes-dislikes we have as individuals.

When you have a goal in mind, there are multiple ways of achieving it, right? You picked up this book with a simple goal of finding a way to lose those inches. But what if I tell you , your weight is not the enemy. The enemy is your unhealthy lifestyle.

And that the solution is also not somewhere far away, it's around you, and within you, all you will need is the simple understanding of your body and its connection with mother nature.

I come from the academic background of medicine and sciences and I found my passion in the understanding of the best form of natural medicine available to us, i.e. food.

My specialization lies in food and nutrition. I believe in the saying, "when your diet is wrong, medicine is of no use but when your diet is right, medicine is of no need".

The issue of obesity has become highly prevalent in India, a staggering 40% of our population is obese and is slowly moving towards a life with serious health risks.

A few years ago I was one of these 40% people too. I had no clue that this weight was not just a constant trigger to my body image but also a road to a disease ridden life. One day a man at a clothing store replied this when I asked him to show me a dress for a family function. He said, "Ma'am aap ke size ki yahan koi dress nahi hai '', there is no dress at our store that can fit your size. This is where the gravity of my situation hit me. It's not the condescending remark that the salesperson made on my size but at that time I realized it's not just about the fat shaming, it's my health and myself that I was putting at stake. Since then I researched the topic attempting to understand the severity and the problem of obesity specifically in the context of our country. And I found that what our grandparents knew so well, the current time somehow erased it all from our heads. The answer to our weight problem is not in any medicine, not in a supplement, not an exercise but it's everything that comprises our lifestyle.

Remember, "what you eat you become". Sure, you can understand this in terms of food but it extends way beyond that. When you consume stress, when you consume junk food, when you consume laziness, you slowly become what you eat.

My study led to the discovery of 5 golden rules that are a game-changer when it comes to healthifying and weight loss and I'll be sharing them with you in this book.

I never profess anything that pushes you to go to extremes just lose the inches, my simple mantra is, the closer you are to the natural order of things, the better your body heals, feels and becomes.

The problem is not exactly obesity, it's just a symptom, the actual issue to address is your unhealthy habits and lifestyle that is causing this symptom to be there. It's a symptom that you can easily see, that's why it worries you but there are so many symptoms that lay hidden, slowly destroying your body from inside. Therefore my goal is to teach you to fight the unhealthy lifestyle and everything else including your weight will rightly fall into place. In this book we will discuss the natural, easy and fun way for you to lose weight. A plan that is 100% backed by scientific knowledge and a lifestyle that is not just for weight loss but to bring out a new healthy, more confident, 'you'.

Chapter 1

WHAT IS THE WEIGHT PROBLEM?

The problem with our current generation is that we look at everything as an isolated event, an event occurring independent of other factors. This is also the reason why people assume that one isolated adjustment in their habits will create a holistic change in their entire life and moreover it will be permanent. When you have a problem you have to address it keeping in mind the multiplicity of factors that are involved in the occurrence of it. Einstein once said, "The definition of insanity is doing the same thing over and over and expecting different results." Our lifestyle screams of foods that are disease causing, nutrition deficient; of lifestyle that is sedentary and affected by volumes of stress. When the inputs are all wrong how do we expect for our bodies to not show the respective results? When you put yourself on a crash diet or you try to avoid one food and replace it with another, you are not addressing the issue at its root. All you are doing is playing hide and seek with your problem. It will hide for some time but in the next turn will seek you back again. Consider this, if you are building a home, you are extremely careful of the foundation. The strength and durability of its material becomes a priority because that is what will hold the entire structure together. But let's say the foundation was somehow not built strong enough and now there are problems of seepage, molds and cracks in the walls. In this situation would you make up for it by just painting the walls outside? No right, because it won't make a difference. What is rotting inside will one day cause the whole structure to fall. The same is true for the body, for our mind and their connection with each other. Our bodies are excellent mirrors of our internal conditions. Your body is not biased against you to put on extra weight and cause trouble for you with it. Your mind doesn't like it when people fat shame you and crush your self-confidence. There is something going on inside that is causing your body to behave and shape in a certain manner. And this is what you need to address first in order to get back to your optimum weight and health.

What determines our weight?

According to the Centers for Disease Control and Prevention, Obesity is a complex disease that occurs when an individual's weight is higher than what is considered healthy for his or her height. Many factors can contribute to excess weight gain including eating patterns, physical activity levels, sleep routines. Social & psychological determinants, genetics,and certain medications. Not every person who is overweight is obese. However both obesity and overweight are defined as abnormal or excessive fat accumulation that may impair health.

What does it mean to gain weight?

Have I become fat?, is both a subjective and an objective observation. What I mean by this is till the time, you do not measure your body weight against a standard set by scientific research, your idea of being overweight can be subjective. For example, a person who expects to be size zero their perception of weight gain might be different from someone who has put on apparently visible belly fat. Both think they are overweight but in both cases the medical and health implications are different. This is why there are certain measures and standards that are designed to bring objectivity into weight classification. Moreover being overweight and being obese are also two different things. Being overweight is a condition where an individual's weight exceeds the healthy limits of weight for a given height. It is generally defined as having a BMI between 25 and 29.9. Obesity is a more severe condition characterized by an excessive accumulation of body fat. It is typically defined as having a BMI of 30 or higher.

BMI and other metrics are some objective measures used by Doctors to check if you are gaining weight which is higher than the expected limits with respect to your height. These measures are defined as :

- ❖ **Body Mass Index (BMI) :** BMI is a widely used and simple method to assess whether a person is overweight or obese. It's calculated by dividing a person's weight in kilograms by the square of their height in meters (BMI = weight (kg) / height (m^2). The resulting number is then categorized as follows:

- Underweight: BMI less than 18.5
- Normal weight: BMI 18.5 to 24.9
- Overweight: BMI 25 to 29.9
- Obesity (Class I): BMI 30 to 34.9
- Obesity (Class II): BMI 35 to 39.9
- Obesity (Class III): BMI 40 or greater

❖ **Waist Circumference:** Waist circumference measures the size of a person's waist and is an indicator of abdominal obesity, which is associated with increased health risks.

❖ **Waist-to-Hip Ratio (WHR):** WHR is the ratio of the circumference of the waist to the circumference of the hips. A high WHR indicates the distribution of fat in the abdominal region, which is associated with a higher risk of obesity-related health issues.

❖ **Skinfold Thickness:** This method involves measuring the thickness of subcutaneous fat at various points on the body using skinfold calipers.

The most common method used is BMI but it doesn't take a lot of important factors into account. So, while deciding on your weight classification you can first take a general idea by using online BMI calculators or doing the calculation on your own and then you can confirm it by visiting a doctor.

Hereon the text is dedicated to my beloved readers who are looking for a solution to 'How To Lose Weight Fast'. Worry not, I am here to bring easy and natural solutions that will not be hard on your pocket, time, your body and mind. I will try best to take you to the root cause of your problems, so that you understand the mechanism behind weight gain and loss. I am here to empower you with knowledge that will guide you throughout your life and will help you to rely on your own intellect to make mindful lifestyle choices. Let's begin!

It's not you It's a phenomenon

"In recent decades, our world is facing a group of health conditions nicknamed 'The New World Syndrome ' emerging from the increasing sedentary lifestyles, social and dietary changes", as per the International Journal of Health Sciences & Research. A recent World Health Organisation (WHO) report estimates that the prevalence of obesity has more than doubled globally. More than 1.9 billion adults above 18 years were overweight and among them, over 600 million were obese.

Lancet publishes that, "Abdominal obesity was found to be more prevalent amongst the women in India putting them at an increased risk of metabolic complications and non-communicable diseases."

According to Express, "The most popular google search is, 'how to lose weight fast', with 486,000 asking Google this question each year." "Surprisingly, a large number of people also want to know how to gain weight, with 79,200 people a year asking Google this question." There are multiple reasons for this phenomenon to take shape worldwide and in our country as well.

"For the past few decades, India saw a growing preference among Indians for western food, with modernisation, urbanization, and economic development," said a Government report. *Urbanization and increasing disposable incomes have led to significant changes in dietary habits. Traditional diets that were once rich in whole grains, fruits, and vegetables are being replaced by calorie-dense and nutrition-poor options.* A phenomenon has taken shape where Indians are moving away from their traditional and local cuisine to the marketed items brought to them by urbanization. There is also a marketed belief and a commercial edge that these consumer products have over the traditional indian snacks. "The report attempted to bring out the uniqueness and scientific character of traditional Indian foods and contrasted them against global cuisines. Contrary to popular belief it was found that Indian food, including snacks, drinks, accompaniments, and sweets, has fewer calories than its non-traditional counterparts." But thanks to aggressive marketing and advertising the foods that are over the limits energy dense and high in sugars and salts, are sold to us as the healthiest options in the market.

In addition to this there are other factors that are equally responsible for turning obesity into a phenomenon especially in India.

❖ **Sedentary Lifestyle:** As India undergoes rapid urbanization, more people are engaged in sedentary occupations and lead less physically active lives. Increased screen time, longer commutes, and a lack of physical activity are contributing to obesity.

- ❖ **Lack of Awareness:** Many individuals and families in India may not have access to or awareness of proper nutrition and healthy eating habits. This lack of awareness can lead to poor dietary choices.
- ❖ **Genetic Factors:** Genetic factors can play a role in an individual's susceptibility to obesity, and some people may be more prone to gaining weight.
- ❖ **Socioeconomic Factors:** Obesity is often associated with socioeconomic status. In India, as in many other countries, lower-income groups may have limited access to nutritious foods and health care, which can contribute to obesity.
- ❖ **Cultural Factors:** Traditional celebrations and cultural norms in India often involve the consumption of rich, calorie-dense foods. This can contribute to overeating during festivals and special occasions.
- ❖ **Lack of Physical Education:** Inadequate emphasis on physical education in schools and a reduction in recreational spaces can limit opportunities for physical activity, particularly among children and adolescents.
- ❖ **Stress and Mental Health:** Stress and mental health issues can lead to emotional eating and weight gain, as individuals may use food as a coping mechanism.
- ❖ **Healthcare Challenges:** Limited access to healthcare and a lack of effective public health campaigns may hinder efforts to combat obesity and promote healthy lifestyles.

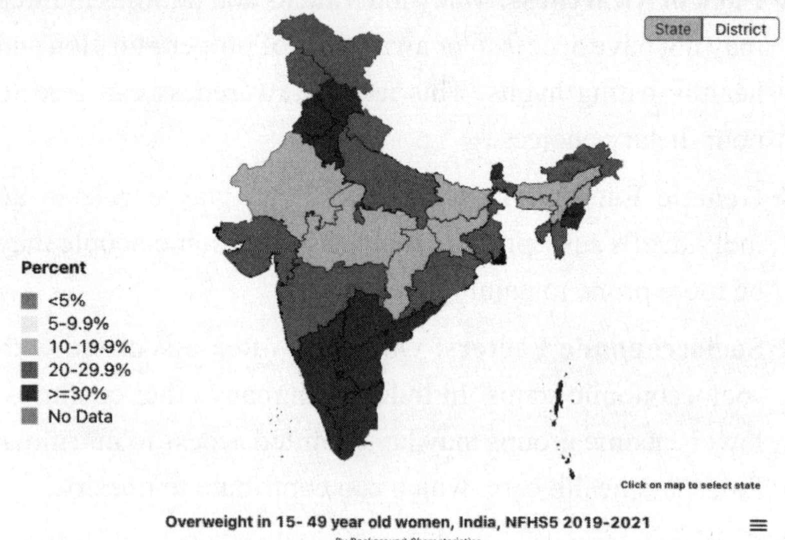

Where to begin with weight loss?

Our body has five major nutritional components that it relies upon to survive and work efficiently : fats, carbohydrates, proteins, vitamins and minerals. The balance of these nutritional components create a healthy body and imbalance in the same creates an unhealthy body. Human body gains weight when it accumulates excess energy in the form of fat. This occurs when a person consumes more calories (energy) through food and beverages than their body expends through metabolic processes and physical activity.

There are two major ways of reducing weight, one is if you reduce your calorie intake and second if you increase your physical activity. When it comes to cutting down on calories there are many ways with which one can achieve it.

Although each way is different and there is no guarantee that they are safe for unprescribed use. What are the most common 'nuske', advice, methods that you have heard from people around you to achieve weight loss? I think the number one would be joining a gym, second would be some sort of a diet and third would be dropping certain foods. As per the data from the National Health and Nutrition Examination Survey USA, Among adolescents who tried to lose weight, the most commonly reported ways were exercising (83.5%); drinking a lot of water (52.3%); eating less (48.6%); eating less junk food or fast food (44.7%); and eating more fruits, vegetables, and salads (44.6%). These ways are actually effective but without knowing the right mix of methods with the right knowledge of your body's constituency, you cannot make these methods work for the long run.

So the most fundamental thing you can understand is the simple equation of weight loss

No. of calories taken < No. of calories burnt

To understand the working of this equation, one needs to monitor the calorie intake and calories burnt in a day. So, let's assess the efficiency of this traditional method of calories monitoring.

Role of Calories monitoring in weight loss

Calories are a unit of measurement used to quantify the amount of energy contained in the food and beverages we consume. The energy our bodies require to function comes from the macronutrients in our diet, primarily carbohydrates, proteins, and fats. When we eat and digest food, our bodies extract and use the energy stored in these macronutrients to fuel various physiological processes, including maintaining body temperature, supporting physical activity, and powering vital organ functions. However sometimes when our food is densely packed with energy and there is not much of it that we expend, the extra energy gets stored as fat in the body. This fat accumulates in different parts of the body. Once the accumulating fat crosses the far limit of optimum levels, it becomes important to regulate it otherwise it becomes a risk factor making a body vulnerable to diseases. Each food has some calories in it, some are abundant in them, some are deficient.

You can find these Indian Foods in your diet that are Abundant in Calories: Biryani, Butter Chicken, Samosas, Paneer Tikka, Gulab Jamun

You can find these Indian Foods in your diet that are Relatively Deficient in Calories: Daal (Lentils), Vegetable Curry, Tandoori Chicken, Raita, Chapati/Roti

To achieve weight loss, the traditional approach is to calculate and monitor the number of calories you take in a day, so that you do not exceed the far limit. It makes you calculate the calories in every little thing you eat but the problem with this route is that the simple act of eating, which is the most fundamental activity of our daily life, becomes too mechanical and too calculative. It is almost equivalent to punishing yourself each and every moment of your life. Food is one of the joys in our life and no one should have to calculate it as a mathematical puzzle. However satisfying and active this process might seem in the beginning but slowly it will wear you out of your energy, your passion and dedication towards 'healthyfying' your life. Something that you cannot continue for your entire life will show results only temporarily. Weight gain doesn't only happen because you exceed your calorie intake everyday or you do not burn your calories everyday, it happens because the food you are putting inside your gut is equivalent to garbage for your body. It does not get what it wants from the food you are eating, therefore it craves for quick energy fixes that you consume as junk food. I understand that fast food and junk food is so tasty and no party can be without them. But what if I tell you that for weight loss you don't have to quit on tasty food and that there is an alternative that you can choose, which will not only help you to lose weight but will transform your body-mind inside out.

Thus weight loss with calorie monitoring may temporarily show results but it will bring you back to the same scales once you let go of the calculations.

Tuning down to a diet that is deficient in calories is important but it is necessary to include other aspects with it too.

Role of Exercise in weight loss

As we discussed, the other side of the equation of weight loss is exercise. A similar monitory of calories burnt is advised for weight loss as well. But this is an oversimplified explanation of a much deeper concept. It appears simple to people that if you exercise more the more you'll burn the extra calories. Afterall, the most common answer to weight loss was found getting to the gym everyday. At the end of the day they promise to get you a slim and fit body. Imagine you have a room that is full of small basketballs. You go into it everyday and work to remove a few balls from inside of it. Gradually the room will empty and become clean again. But now consider this, let's say you take out 10 balls everyday from that room in the morning and in the evening add 10 balls back to the room again. Will the room ever get empty if things continue like this? No, right? Because in order for the room to empty again, you have to work everyday to remove the balls and make sure that you are not adding more than or even equivalent to what you are removing from the room. Now imagine this, while working to remove those balls, your body feels extremely tired and mind feels the agony of doing something it hates. Won't your energy levels and the quality of your work decline with each day? Similarly it is with our bodies as well. You are working to burn 'x' amount of calories through exercise but you are adding equivalent or more than what you are burning everyday. On top of that some people get into intensive exercises without considering the level of their staminas and fitness. Moreover some people choose physical activities that they do not enjoy at all, and this adds to the pressure on both mind and body. No matter how much you exercise, if you don't have the understanding and the full picture of it, you will end up with the same saturated room over and over again. And the more effort you put in to do the futile cleaning, the worse it will become for you and your body. As the process will take up a lot of your mental and physical energy.

A recent research published by NIH in its journal stated, "Patients wishing to lose weight should participate in physical activity and caloric restriction to improve the chances of weight loss. Overall clinicians should attempt to encourage participants to adhere to ET programs over the long-term regardless of the amount of weight loss achieved, as CV benefits are readily achieved in the absence of weight loss."

What does this suggest? The research basically says that only a combined effort made on caloric reduction and physical activity will help you achieve weight loss. Doing just either of them will not get you long lasting and effective results as weight loss is a multi sided equation. Moreover it is stated that physical activity is especially effective when you exercise what you enjoy.

So, let's also discuss what type of exercise one should do on a daily basis. Researchers often get asked what is the best exercise and how much exercise one should do. The researchers replied, "At the end of the day, the best exercise is one you enjoy and can sustain over time." So, if you enjoy 30 minutes of brisk walking do that, if you enjoy playing table tennis or any other sport do that. The only motive behind it should be to get your body moving and getting it to be healthier. Always remember weight is not a problem in itself, it is a symptom of what all is going wrong inside. So, stress, wrong diet choices, imbalanced work-life are all the things that are going wrong inside that have created a problem of weight and fat for you. Therefore, choose an exercise that doesn't feel like punishment to you. Choose something that allows you to break that monotony of everyday life and something that reminds you to be alive again.

This strategy works two ways, one it helps you to burn off calories and second it helps you to manage everyday stress in a better way.

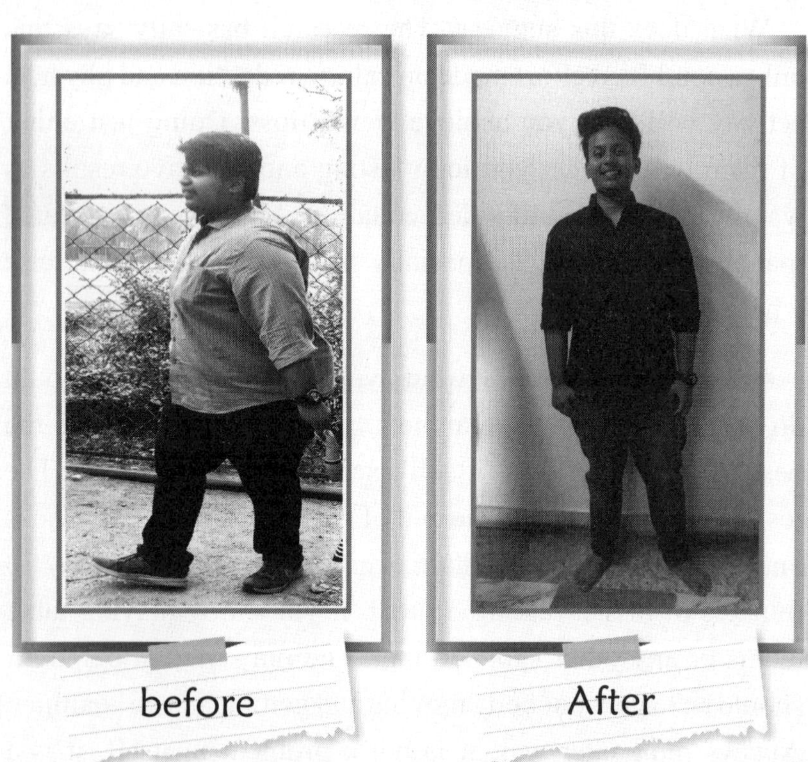

Chapter - 2

5 GOLDEN RULES TO WEIGHT LOSS

Our lives are mostly out of sync from the natural order, today. Everyone is a prey to a busy life schedule, requiring constant work so much so that there is hardly any time left to care for our own bodies and minds.

Our time commitments are all over the place. It is really hard to achieve work-life balance in today's times because each one of us wants to succeed in life and do good. This intensity of ambition and a drive to move ahead in life, is a good thing for our professional lives but it leaves behind your health and wellbeing hanging on the shelf. So what are the changes we can adopt that can very easily change the course of your life, health and of course help you lose body weight.

Let's dive deeper into these five golden rules.

1. Prioritize Your Sleep:

Adequate sleep is fundamental for physical and mental well-being. Poor sleep can disrupt hormones that regulate appetite and lead to overeating. "Sleep deprivation is associated with an increased risk of obesity, a poor lipid–lipoprotein profile, type 2 diabetes mellitus (DM), hypertension and other cardiovascular diseases (CVD). The National Health and Nutrition Examination Survey (NHANES) showed significantly higher rates of obesity in adults who reported an average of less than 7 h a night of sleep". Sleep deprivation can contribute to obesity by increasing appetite through hormonal imbalances, promoting cravings for high-calorie foods, reducing energy expenditure and exercise motivation, disrupting glucose metabolism and promoting insulin resistance, raising stress levels and cortisol release, disturbing circadian rhythms and eating patterns, encouraging late-night, unhealthy eating, and impairing decision-making and self-control. These factors collectively create an environment conducive to weight gain and can lead to obesity when sleep deprivation becomes chronic. This was the summary of impacts of sleep deprivation in medical language.But let me explain it to you simply. See, sleeping for 7-8 hours evernight is extremely essential for our bodies. However, it is more important that you get this 7-8 hours of sleep at the right time. What do I mean by the right time? It refers to the sleep schedule that allows you to have deep sleep i.s. REM sleep. Deep sleep is where our bodies actually replenish, recover, and rejuvenate. The right time to sleep is around 10:00 PM/10:30 PM to 6:00 AM/6:30 AM. Whenever you go to bed beyond 10:30 PM at night our body begins to undergo hormonal fluctuations which are not healthy at all. Primary example of this is the synthesis of higher levels of cortisol by adrenal glands in the body, which impacts almost all the areas of our normal functioning. Higher levels of cortisol can raise blood sugar levels, weaken the immune system, cause weight gain (especially around the abdomen), lead to muscle loss, reduce bone density, and increase the risk of heart problems and mental health issues like anxiety and depression. Cortisol can also disrupt sleep patterns and skin health, as well as affect the digestive system. Managing stress and maintaining a healthy lifestyle are important to regulate cortisol levels and prevent these potential negative effects on the body.

When you don't get enough sleep, your body produces more of a hormone called ghrelin, which makes you feel hungry. It also reduces the production of another hormone called leptin, which tells your brain that you're full. So, when you're sleep-deprived, you tend to feel hungrier and might eat more. Lack of sleep can make you crave unhealthy, high-calorie, and sugary foods. You're more likely to reach for snacks and junk food when you're tired, which can lead to weight gain.When you're tired, you have less energy for physical activity and exercise. This can make it harder to burn calories and lose weight because you might not feel like being active. Poor sleep can slow down your metabolism, which is how your body burns calories. A slower metabolism means you burn fewer calories, making it more challenging to lose weight.

Therefore prioritizing adequate and quality sleep is crucial for maintaining a healthy weight and overall well-being. Here's how to prioritize your sleep:

- Aim for 7-8 hours of quality sleep per night.
- Create a consistent sleep schedule by going to bed and waking up at the same time each day.
- Establish a relaxing bedtime routine to signal to your body that it's time to wind down.
- Keep your sleep environment comfortable, dark, and quiet.
- Avoid screens (phones, computers, TVs) at least an hour before bedtime, as the blue light emitted can interfere with your sleep.

2. Drink 3-4 Liters of Water Every Day:

"Most beverages can support hydration, but water is unique in doing this without also adding sugars or many other compounds into the diet," states the NIH paper. Staying well-hydrated is important for overall health and can also support weight loss. Drinking 3-4 liters of water daily can support weight management in various ways. Adequate hydration can boost metabolic rate and promote a sense of fullness, potentially reducing calorie intake during meals. Water is a calorie-free beverage and can replace high-calorie or sugary drinks, helping to lower overall daily calorie consumption. Proper hydration aids digestion, reducing the likelihood of digestive discomfort that might lead to unhealthy eating habits. Additionally, staying well-hydrated can enhance exercise performance, facilitating more effective calorie burning during physical activity. While water is a valuable component of a healthy lifestyle, it's important to remember that weight management involves a combination of factors, including diet, exercise, and overall lifestyle choices, and excessive water consumption should be avoided. Here's how to incorporate more water into your daily routine:

- Carry a reusable water bottle with you to remind yourself to drink regularly.
- Drink a glass of water before meals to help control your appetite.
- Infuse your water with slices of fruits, vegetables, or herbs for added flavor.
- Avoid sugary drinks, as they can add unnecessary calories to your diet.

3. Monitor Your Weight Regularly:

A study published in the NIH journal stated, "Weighing everyday led to greater adoption of weight control behaviors and produced greater weight loss compared to weighing most days of the week. This further indicates daily weighing as an effective weight loss tool." A similar study done by Stanford University suggested, " No matter which weight loss tactic you choose, you're typically more successful if you track your progress with digital health tools." These are the lines from Obesity action forum, "The bottom line is that no matter how you do it, self-monitoring should be an important part of your weight-loss, weight maintenance or healthy lifestyle change." Keeping track of your weight can help you stay accountable and make adjustments to your lifestyle as needed.

Monitoring your weight regularly is a valuable tool on your weight loss journey. It fosters accountability, provides feedback on your efforts, and can serve as motivation to stay committed to your goals. It also helps you detect issues early, make informed adjustments to your diet and exercise routine, and deter overeating. By tracking your weight trends over time, you can set realistic goals and develop strategies to overcome plateaus. However, it's essential to approach weight monitoring with a healthy perspective, recognizing that weight can fluctuate naturally and using it as one of several metrics to assess progress. Consulting with a healthcare professional or dietitian can offer personalized guidance for effective and safe weight loss.

Here are some tips for weight monitoring:

- Weigh yourself at the same time of day, preferably in the morning, before eating or drinking.
- Use the same scale each time for consistency.
- Record your weight in a journal or on a mobile app to track your progress over time.
- Remember that weight can naturally fluctuate, so focus on trends over several weeks rather than day-to-day changes.

4. Reduce Stress in Life:

These are the quoted statements from a research published by Stanford University. "It may sound surprising, but stress actually plays a large role in your waistline and how easily you can lose weight. For example, multiple studies show how stress and lack of sleep can lead to an increase in your cortisol levels (the stress hormone). Having higher levels of cortisol in your body can cause you to:

- feel hungrier; and
- crave foods that have a lot of sugar, calories, and fat.

Higher cortisol levels can also cause people to build up fat around their bellies.

Learning to reduce stress through exercise and meditation—while also being more mindful about food—can have a large impact on your well-being and help you keep weight off in the long-term."

Chronic stress can contribute to weight gain and overall health problems. Reducing stress in your life can be a powerful ally in your weight loss journey. Stress triggers the release of cortisol, a hormone associated with fat storage, and can lead to emotional eating, poor sleep, and impaired decision-making when it comes to diet and exercise. Lowering stress levels can positively impact hormonal balance, increase energy levels, and improve your ability to make healthier choices. Stress-reduction techniques, such as meditation and mindfulness, can foster emotional well-being and long-term sustainability in your weight loss efforts. By managing stress, you not only promote weight loss but also support your overall health and well-being.

To reduce stress:

- Practice relaxation techniques such as deep breathing, meditation, or yoga.
- Identify stressors in your life and develop strategies to manage or reduce them.
- Get regular exercise, as physical activity can help relieve stress and improve mood.
- Make time for hobbies and activities you enjoy to help you unwind.

5. Dinner Before 7:

There have been several studies that have proven the above-stated fact. This practice helps reduce weight loss and triggers the metabolism. This practice automatically leads to Intermittent Fasting. During Fasting, the body fulfills its energy demands from the stored body fat instead of the glucose in the fed state. Eating dinner earlier in the evening can have several benefits for your health and weight management. Having dinner before 7 p.m. can be a beneficial practice for weight loss. It promotes better digestion before bedtime, reduces the likelihood of late-night snacking on calorie-dense foods, and helps maintain stable blood sugar levels. It encourages increased physical activity after dinner, aligns with the body's natural circadian rhythm for balanced appetite hormones, and provides a longer fasting period before breakfast, potentially supporting fat burning and improved insulin sensitivity. Moreover, it can enhance sleep quality, which plays a crucial role in regulating hormones related to appetite and metabolism.

- It gives your body more time to digest the food before you go to bed, reducing the risk of acid reflux and indigestion.
- Eating earlier can help regulate your circadian rhythm and improve sleep quality.
- You're less likely to consume excess calories before bedtime, which can contribute to weight gain.

Incorporating a comprehensive approach to weight loss, which includes getting 7-8 hours of sleep, having dinner before 7 p.m., monitoring weight regularly, reducing stress, and drinking 3-4 liters of water every day, in conjunction with a well-balanced diet plan, can significantly support your weight loss journey. As I told you before as well, overweight and obesity are just symptoms of a lifestyle dysfunctionality that is working behind the scenes. Once you correct these fundamental habits in your life, not just your weight but all other things will balance themselves as a result. Sufficient sleep aids in hormonal balance and appetite control, while an earlier dinner can improve digestion and prevent late-night snacking. Regular weight monitoring offers feedback and motivation, while stress reduction techniques and hydration promote healthier choices and overall well-being.

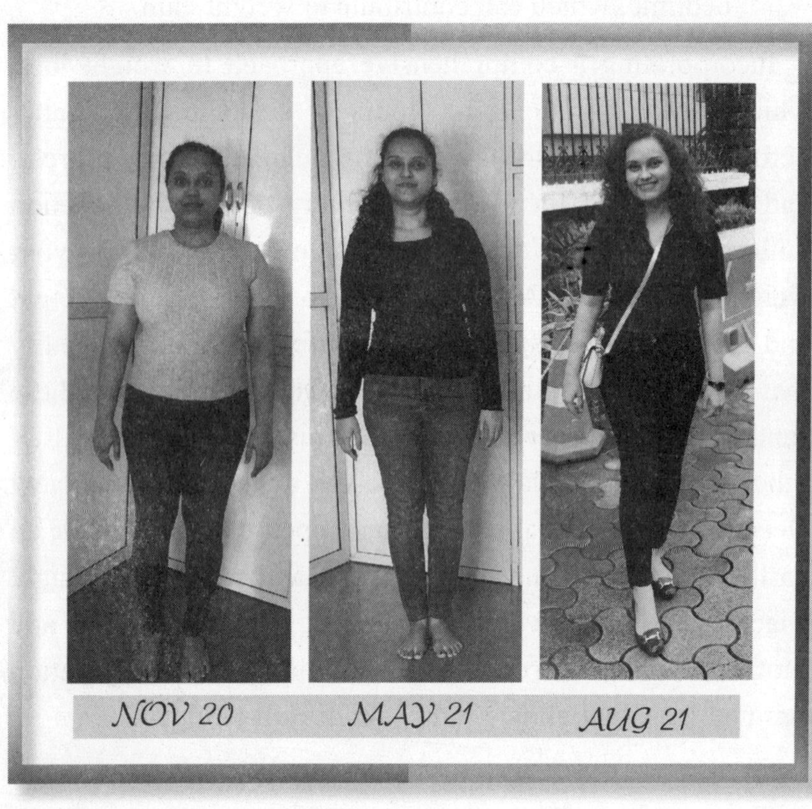
NOV 20
MAY 21
AUG 21

Chapter 3 :

WHAT MAKES A GOOD DIET FOR WEIGHT LOSS?

As promised in the introduction to this book, I am now gonna start with the real work now. So as we have already established, there are some essentials to weight loss and diet forms the most important component of this journey.

Introduction

The five golden rules that we learnt about in the last chapter deal primarily with the lifestyle changes that are necessary to achieve weight loss. However lifestyle is one part of this equation and the other part relies heavily on diet. Before we get into the details, let's try to answer, what is diet? A diet encompasses all the nutritional choices and eating habits that make up an individual's daily or long-term eating pattern. Diets can vary widely from person to person and can be influenced by cultural, personal, health, and ethical factors. Diets can also be designed for specific purposes, such as weight management, improving overall health, addressing medical conditions, or adhering to dietary restrictions or preferences.

Some common types of diet that you might have heard of are balanced diet, keto, gluten-free and vegan diet.

Most people often use the concept of diet and fasting interchangeably. However the word 'Dieting' actually refers to a practice of intentionally regulating one's food and caloric intake in order to achieve specific health, fitness, or weight-related goals. It is an action plan of choosing diet & nutrition in a way that can help you direct your body and mind in a certain way. It doesn't automatically refer to fasting or starving yourself of food and liquids.

Contrary to the popular beliefs, good nutrition can help one to drop inches as it works very effectively in hitting the root cause of being overweight. Food is a form of natural medicine to our body. If our diet is right we shall never require to take any other medications in our life.

Good nutrition satiates your body and reduces cravings for other foods or liquids. Actually, the major reason behind cravings is the lack of nutrition which results in your body asking for quick fixes in the form of heavy sugars and salts. The second reason is that a good diet is packed with fiber which gives bulk to our food, reducing the requirement of eating more. Moreover roughage in the fiber helps clean out our digestive system. Furthermore, foods rich in nutrients require increased chewing, which in turn slows your eating pace, and makes you more mindful of the action of eating. As a result, your body has a chance to send the signals to the brain that let you know when you're full. Now that we know how important good nutrition is for our proper functioning and aiding in weight loss, let's try to understand what exactly is a good diet.

A good diet comprises three components, nutrition, local availability and seasonality. This further definition is given by the NIH journal based on a study, "Healthy diets, arising either by tradition or design, share many common features and generally align with the WHO Global Action Plan for the Prevention and Control of Noncommunicable Diseases. In comparison with a Western diet, these healthier alternatives are higher in plant-based foods, including fresh fruits and vegetables, whole grains, legumes, seeds, and nuts and lower in animal-based foods, particularly fatty and processed meats." Therefore any food that is seasonal, locally sourced and holds a good nutritional value is a good food. Beyond this a good diet even brings into consideration the portion size of each nutrient.

For this there is a very simple method called **the plate method.**

Take a plate and fill half the plate with **vegetables**, they can be cooked or tossed as a salad.

Fill a quarter of the plate with **lean protein** eg. meat, seafood, poultry, eggs, dairy, legumes, tofu.

Fill the remaining quarter of the plate with **complex carbohydrates**, eg. whole grains.

"According to the Dietary Guidelines for Americans 2020–2025, a healthy eating plan,

- Will always contain fruits, vegetables, whole grains, milk and milk products (low-fat)
- Includes a variety of protein foods such as seafood, lean meats and poultry, eggs, legumes (beans and peas), soy products, nuts, and seeds.
- Is low in added sugars, sodium, saturated fats, trans fats, and cholesterol.
- Stays within your daily calorie needs

Components of a good diet for weight loss:

Based on the plate method the three most important components of your meal are vegetables, proteins and carbohydrates. So, let's learn more about these in this section.

Vegetables are valuable for weight loss because their calorie content is low, they contain high fiber, veggies are rich in water content, and are nutritionally dense. Eating vegetables in the right portion size besides providing essential vitamins and minerals, gives a feeling of fullness which in turn helps control cravings. Since their calorie density is low, you can add a variety of veggies to your diet without worrying about the weight gain from eating them. However, it's essential to maintain portion control and choose healthy preparation methods to maximize their benefits for weight loss as well as your overall health.

Protein is one of the most important macronutrients as it is the building block of our body starting from the cellular level. Our blood, skin, hair, nails, bones and muscles everything is made up of protein. Protein also makes it possible for our bodily functions like growth, maintenance, repair, digestion, metabolism, immunity etc. conduct and occur effectively. Once protein fulfills its function, it either gets stored as fat in the body or gets excreted in the form of waste. Thus like any other macronutrient both its deficiency and abundance creates a problem for the body. When you take sufficient protein your body has enough fuel to run its functions properly without any problem. But if you exceed the limits of protein intake, your body will store it as fat resulting in weight gain. This is why only a quarter of your plate should be taken as protein following your preference for either plant based or animal based protein.

So now that we have fairly discussed the importance and characteristics of good diet & nutrition, let's learn to incorporate the important components we discussed above into the diet plan especially targeted at weight loss. My diet plan consists of three usual meals, breakfast, lunch and dinner. Besides the usual there are mid-time snacks and drinks that I offer as unique additions to my diet plan. These additions are not here just so that my diet plan stands out from the rest but the logic behind mid-time drink is highly rooted in the science of weight loss and nutrition. Mid-time snacks allow our body to have a boost of nutrition before actually sitting for the big three meals. As a result we do not eat more than required and through healthy snacking, we get that extra dose of nutrition as well. I always say that, contrary to popular belief, eating less is not the answer to weight loss, the answer is eating right and eating at the right time.

Basic diet plan for a day

❖ **This is how your meals should be scheduled for the entire day.**

Morning drink- 7-7:30

Breakfast 8-8:30

Mid Morning snack-10-10:30

Lunch-1-1:30

Evening drink + seeds

Dinner-7-7:30

Night drink-8:30-9:00

Morning tea/Night tea-

One of the most important steps that I followed in my weight loss routine was the teas that I had. This single step gave me an edge over the standard weight loss practices that are usually followed. When 'a 110 kilos me' was working towards getting to my normal BMI which was around 60 kilos, there was a period when my body entered a state of weight loss plateau. The fat that was stuck inside was not able to leave the body with normal dietary changes and exercises, this is when the different tea concoctions that I made and consumed pushed the progress further. Sometimes when we are in the process of losing weight, the body enters a plateau stage. This is a state where no matter how much diet and exercise you regulate and experiment with, your body refuses to change any further. This is when tea concoctions help to break the inertia and ease weight loss even further. The teas give superb inch loss especially around the belly, thighs and hip area which are mostly problematic areas for most people trying to lose weight. The teas that I am going to share with you in this chapter are the ones that I myself have used during my weight loss journey and the ones that I truly believe in.You can choose any two of them and continue the same for 15 days after which you swap it with a new one. There was research done on mice, who were given green tea along with a high fat diet. According to this paper published by Penn State, "mice on a high-fat diet that consumed decaffeinated green tea extract and exercised regularly experienced sharp reductions in final body weight and significant improvements in health, researchers suggested that similar results could be realized by people as well.

After 16 weeks, high-fat-fed mice that exercised regularly and ingested green tea extract showed an average body mass reduction of 27.1 percent and an average abdominal fat mass reduction of 36.6 percent."

There are more studies being conducted in order to have a deeper understanding of the working of such natural teas for weight loss in humans. However there is an existing consensus on some additional benefits that these natural teas offer :

❖ **Metabolism Boost:** Some teas, especially green tea, contain compounds like catechins and caffeine that can increase metabolism. This can help the body burn more calories, supporting weight loss when combined with a balanced diet and regular exercise.

- ❖ **Reduced Appetite:** Certain teas have been linked to appetite suppression. This can be helpful in managing weight by potentially reducing the intake of unnecessary calories throughout the day.
- ❖ **Improved Digestion:** Herbal teas aid digestion, preventing bloating and indigestion, which can indirectly support weight management.
- ❖ **Antioxidants:** Many teas are rich in antioxidants, which can support overall health. Antioxidants can help in reducing inflammation and supporting the body's natural detoxification processes, potentially aiding weight loss efforts.
- ❖ **Hydration:** Staying hydrated is essential for overall health and can support weight loss by keeping the body functioning optimally. Tea, when consumed without added sugars or milk, can contribute to daily hydration goals.

The efficacy of teas, though not very prominently and deeply studied by modern science, has been present in our traditional knowledge forever.

Now let's make some tasty and healthy teas with these recipes

7 Tea options

The preparation for each tea is similar however the

ingredients and their portion will differ. The same are mentioned alongside each tea option.

Preparation-

Step 1- Add 1 liter of water to a pan if you are making morning tea and 1 glass of water if you are making night tea.

Step 2- Add the required ingredients according to their portion sizes mentioned below.

Step 3- Cover with a lid and let it come to a boil

Step 4- Strain the tea and drink while warm on an empty stomach.

In the case of morning tea you can have the remaining tea water throughout the day after warming it each time.

1. Jeera tea- Fennel tea- Use 2 tbsp fennel
2. Cinnamon tea- Use 2 cinnamon sticks. Add lemon water after it cools to lukewarm temperature.
3. Coriander- Use 2 tbsp dry coriander seeds.
4. Turmeric tea- Use ¼ tbsp black pepper powder, 2 cinnamon stick, 1 tbsp grated ginger, 1 tbsp grated turmeric root or 2-3 pinch of turmeric powder.
5. Ajwain tea- Use 1/4th tbsp ajwain seeds
6. Tej patta tea- Use 2 tej patta/bay leaves
7. Star Anise Tea- 1 cinnamon stick, 1 star anise, 1 black cardamom

Breakfast-

Breakfast is the most important meal of the day and one should never skip this. I can understand that our schedules as working men/women, a student, or a busy housewife doesn't leave us with any time for self-care but skipping your meals, especially breakfast, creates a lot of problems for your body. The literal meaning of 'breakfast' in itself is breaking your fast. If you have breakfast early around 8:00-8:30 AM, you will notice a change in the energy levels of your body. Your body once refueled with a good diet as your morning meal will help you focus better on your work and function efficiently throughout the day. On the contrary, a late breakfast will always cause you to be in a lethargy and irritated mood for the rest of your day. So, make sure you have your breakfast within 1-2 hours of waking up from your sleep. Given the nature of our modern lives I understand that the steps involved in getting this morning meal to your stomach sounds too heavy. This is why I suggest that you plan ahead for the morning meal or cook it at night so that the only thing you have to do in the morning is just eat your food. If you want to have a fresh meal in the morning, you can at least get the preparations done at night, so that cooking in the morning becomes easier and faster.

I believe that no matter how much I tell you about the importance of breakfast, you will only internalize once you understand the science behind its role for your health and weight loss and also what actually happens when you skip your first meal of the day.

Eating breakfast in the morning jumpstarts your metabolism, the process by which your body burns calories for energy. When you skip breakfast, your body may enter a state of energy conservation, slowing down your metabolism, which can make it harder to burn calories throughout the day. Having a nutritious breakfast regulates your appetite and reduces the likelihood of overeating later in the day. When you skip breakfast, you may become hungrier as the day goes on, making it more likely that you'll consume larger portions and snack on high-calorie foods.Eating breakfast stabilizes your blood sugar levels, which can prevent energy crashes and cravings for sugary or high-calorie snacks. A balanced breakfast that includes fiber, protein, and healthy fats can provide sustained energy and help maintain stable blood sugar levels. When you have a good breakfast, you feel more energized and motivated to engage in physical activity. Regular exercise is an essential component of weight loss, and starting your day with breakfast can set a positive tone for an active lifestyle.

Eating a well-balanced breakfast provides essential nutrients your body needs to function properly. Skipping breakfast may lead to nutrient deficiencies, which can affect your overall health and potentially lead to weight gain. A healthy breakfast can enhance your cognitive function, helping you make better food choices throughout the day. This can lead to more mindful eating and reduced consumption of unhealthy, high-calorie foods.

While I do say that breakfast is an important meal I also say that it is equally important for you to be mindful of what you eat as part of this meal. I do not want you to be eating oil greased paranthas and calorie dense foods in the morning. Then, what should you actually eat? Keeping this in mind, I have created 7 easy breakfast recipes for you which will save you time and provide you all the health and weight loss benefits while still tasting all yummy.

4 recipes -100 words each

1. Paneer sandwich

Saute cumin seeds, green chilli, turmeric and red chilli powder in a pan with desi ghee. To this add chopped onions and then low fat paneer. Saute this for 1-2 minutes and take the pan off the stove. Add the content of the pan as a layer for your sandwich and then put it to grill. Your healthy tasty sandwich is ready. This sandwich is rich in protein and other nutrients which will keep you full for a longer period of time.

2. Besan chilla- Take 1 chopped onion, 1 chopped tomato, half chopped carrot, 1/2 chopped capsicum and to this you can also add any other vegetable of your choice. Mix the vegetables with one bowl of besan. Add salt, chili, hing, cumin seeds as per taste. Then add water to mix the batter but keeping the consistency a little on the thicker side. Grease a pan with oil and pour a small amount of batter on it, spread it evenly to form a chilla shape. Cook with the lid on and flip to cook the other side of the chilla. Serve it with home cooked chutney instead of market ketchup.

Enjoy your tasty breakfast which will not at all cause you to add weight to your body.

3 Moong dal chilla- soak a bowl of whole green gram dal/ moong dal overnight or at least for four hours. Add it to a blender along with chopped ginger, 1 green chili, 1 tbsp cumin seeds, pinch of Hing, salt and a few black peppercorns. Run the blender while adding little water to the mixture. Take out the mixture in a bowl and add a chopped onion to it (you can skip this step in case you do not eat onions). Batter's consistency again should be a little on the thicker side. Grease a pan with oil and pour a small amount of batter on it, spread it evenly to form a chilla shape. Cook with the lid on and flip to cook the other side of the chilla. Serve it with home cooked chutney instead of market ketchup. Enjoy your tasty breakfast which will not at all cause you to add weight to your body.

Mid morning snack

A mid-morning snack is supposed to be taken around 11:00-11:30 in the morning. It can play a valuable role in weight loss for several reasons:

Having a mid-morning snack can help control your appetite and prevent overeating during lunch. When you're too hungry, you may be more likely to consume larger portions or make less healthy choices.

Consuming a healthy snack between breakfast and lunch can help maintain steady blood sugar levels, reducing the likelihood of energy dips and cravings that can lead to unhealthy snacking later in the day.A well-balanced mid-morning snack provides your body with a boost of energy, making you more alert and productive, which can be particularly beneficial for those with active lifestyles. Eating regular, smaller meals and snacks throughout the day can help keep your metabolism active, as your body has a constant supply of energy to burn. Snacking on nutrient-dense options like seasonal and locally available fruits, chickpeas, or boiled eggs can contribute to your daily intake of essential vitamins, minerals, and antioxidants, supporting overall health.

Examples of healthy mid-morning snacks, such as seasonal and locally available options, include:

- **Fresh Fruit:** Sliced apples, oranges, berries, or a banana can provide natural sugars, fiber, and vitamins.
- **Chickpeas (Channa):** Roasted chickpeas are a protein-rich and crunchy snack that can help keep you full and satisfied.
- **Boiled Eggs:** Hard-boiled eggs are an excellent source of protein and healthy fats, which can promote satiety.
- **Greek Yogurt:** Low-fat Greek yogurt with a drizzle of honey and some berries is a high-protein, probiotic-rich snack.
- **Nuts:** A small portion of nuts, like almonds or walnuts, provides healthy fats and protein.
- **Vegetable Sticks:** Carrot, cucumber, and celery sticks with hummus can be a low-calorie, fiber-rich choice.

Lunch plan

- One of the most important things that people usually forget to understand is that eating healthy creates a healthy weight. When you overeat or don't eat as much as is required, it creates problems for the body and this is when it starts acquiring unhealthy weight or starts losing too much. Eating healthy also involves eating meals on time and in sync with our circadian rhythm. Hence, all our meals and their respective timings are very important. Lunch is an important part of our day and sometimes it is not given as much importance as its morning-evening counterparts. However a good and a healthy lunch comes with the following benefits-
- **Energy and Productivity:** Lunch provides a midday energy boost, helping to combat fatigue and maintain productivity throughout the day. It replenishes glycogen stores in the body, ensuring a steady supply of glucose for the brain and muscles.
- **Nutrient Intake:** Lunch is an opportunity to consume essential nutrients, including vitamins, minerals, and macronutrients like carbohydrates, protein, and healthy fats. These nutrients support overall health and well-being.
- **Blood Sugar Regulation:** Eating lunch helps stabilize blood sugar levels, preventing the energy highs and lows associated with skipping meals. This is particularly important for people with conditions like diabetes.

- **Appetite Control:** Having a balanced lunch can prevent excessive hunger later in the day, reducing the likelihood of overeating during dinner or indulging in unhealthy snacks.
- **Weight Management:** Regular meals, including lunch, can contribute to better weight management by helping control portion sizes and reduce impulsive eating.
- **Cognitive Function:** Proper nutrition at lunchtime supports cognitive function, concentration, and memory, which is especially important for students and professionals.
- **Digestive Health:** Eating lunch encourages regular digestion and can help prevent issues like indigestion or acid reflux that might occur if the stomach remains empty for extended periods.
- **Mood and Well-Being:** Consuming a well-rounded lunch can improve mood and reduce feelings of irritability and stress associated with hunger.
- **Social and Cultural Aspects:** Lunch often serves as a social and cultural meal, providing an opportunity to connect with family, friends, or colleagues. These social interactions contribute to emotional well-being.
- A study done on 420 obese people in their daily meal times, stated that people who had their lunch before 3 pm lost more weight than those who had a late lunch. Therefore it is necessary that you have your lunch around 1-1:30 PM in the afternoon. This small step can

take you way ahead in your weight loss journey.

- Here are some interesting, healthy and tasty lunch options for your weight loss.

1. Protein salad

- In a large mixing bowl, combine half a bowl of cooked chickpeas/white chhole. To this add 1 chopped tomato, cucumber, onion, blanched french beans, bell pepper, and fresh herbs like coriander.
- If desired, add roasted peanuts, roasted jeera powder, black pepper powder, chat masala and lemon juice for extra flavor and added benefits.
- Toss everything together until well combined.
- Let the salad sit for about 15-30 minutes to allow the flavors to meld.
- Serve your chickpea protein salad and this amazing tasty protein rich salad.
- protein-rich salads can help preserve lean muscle mass during weight loss. The fiber from vegetables and legumes in the salad aids in digestion and contributes to a feeling of fullness, reducing the likelihood of snacking on unhealthy options between meals. Furthermore, the wide range of vitamins, minerals, and antioxidants from vegetables and fresh herbs in the salad supports overall health and well-being.

Evening snack-

Oftentimes when I am working with my clients in their

journey to weight loss, they bring a common concern to me, CRAVINGS!!!. My clients often come up to me asking for a little snacky reward for all their sacrifice and perseverance on this journey. And to this I often tell them that even though you can't take those marketed snackibles but being healthy and on a weight loss doesn't mean you can't find alternative for healthy snacking. And this is often returned to me with a statement, "so you are saying that I can eat snacks, and it won't harm my health or make me fat?" And my answer is YES!!. I totally understand how difficult it is to not give in to those cravings and have a piece of your favorite chips, chocolates, cakes etc. But I also ask my clients why you think a snack is only that which is found in packets, and is shelved in supermarkets. You create your own tasty-healthy snacks and I'll teach you how. Snacks can be fun, exciting and tasty for us as well, given that the choice of food that we are taking at this time is healthy and carefully crafted to be calorie deficit.

Besides the usual idea of it, my kind of snacks will provide you with the following benefits-

- Control Overeating: Having a small, nutritious snack in the evening can prevent overeating during dinner or late-night snacking. It can help satisfy your hunger and reduce the likelihood of consuming excessive calories.
- Steady Blood Sugar Levels: Eating a balanced evening snack can help stabilize blood sugar levels. When your blood sugar is stable, you're less likely to experience

intense cravings for unhealthy, high-calorie foods.

- Boost Metabolism: Consuming a small, healthy snack can help maintain your metabolism by providing a source of energy. This can prevent your body from going into a "starvation mode," which can slow down your metabolic rate.
- Improve Sleep: A light, nutritious snack before bed can help promote better sleep. Poor sleep has been linked to weight gain and an increased desire for high-calorie, unhealthy foods.
- Nutrient Intake: Evening snacks can be an opportunity to boost your nutrient intake. Including foods rich in vitamins, minerals, and fiber can help ensure you're getting essential nutrients without overindulging.
- Reduce Late-Night Cravings: Having a healthy snack can help satisfy late-night cravings and prevent you from reaching for unhealthy, calorie-dense options.
- Here is one example of a fun alternative I came up with to the market item-
- Granola bar- roast chopped almonds, walnuts, oats together and add jaggery to it. Roast till jaggery melts and mixes well with the seeds. Take a blender and add 8-10 dates to it. Blend well and take the mixture out, to this add the roasted seeds. Mix well with coconut powder, cinnamon powder and a few rose petals. Take a steel container, layer it with a butter paper and press the mixture layer by layer in this container.

Refrigerate the content for 1-2 hours and cut the cake into fine bars.

You can find plenty of more options and recipes on my youtube channel

Dinner -

People often find themselves utterly confused with the complexity of weight loss plans and strategies. So their hope filled question for me is, what is that one thing, that one mantra which if I follow I can lose my extra weight. I tell them that even though weight loss is much more than one hack or a mantra, if you do this one thing right you will see tremendous changes in the way your body functions and definitely in your body weight. The answer lies in the content and timings of your dinner. If you have your dinner at the right time, in the right amount and with the right content, you will surely see changes in your body. Try having a healthy dinner before 7PM at night and I guarantee you will see weight loss as a result.

Research shows that the timing of food intake is an external synchronizer and plays a crucial role in obesity and weight loss treatment. "Breakfast skipping is causally linked to obesity and late lunch (after 15:00 h) hinders weight loss, mainly in those carriers of a genetic variant in Perilipin . Late lunch eating has a deleterious effect on microbiota diversity and composition . Late dinner (within two hours before bedtime) decreases glucose tolerance. Finally, we have described some heritability studies in twins which show that dinner timing is more cultural (0% heritability), and easier to change than breakfast timing which is highly heritable (56%)."

Here are added benefits that come with timely dinners-

1. Eating dinner earlier in the evening can help curb late-night snacking, which is often associated with consuming unhealthy, calorie-dense foods. Late-night snacking can lead to weight gain because the body's metabolism slows down as it prepares for sleep, and excess calories consumed at this time are more likely to be stored as fat.
2. Improved Digestion: Having an early dinner allows for better digestion because your body has more time to process and absorb nutrients before going to bed. This can help prevent indigestion, acid reflux, and discomfort, which can be aggravated by lying down immediately after eating.
3. Better Sleep: Eating too close to bedtime can disrupt sleep as the body works to digest food, potentially leading to discomfort, indigestion, or acid reflux. Poor sleep quality can impact weight loss efforts, as inadequate sleep can lead to increased hunger and reduced willpower.
4. Time-Restricted Eating (TRE): Early dinners are often part of a time-restricted eating (TRE) approach, which limits the window of time during which you can consume food. TRE can help control calorie intake and promote weight loss by creating a consistent daily fasting period. For example, if you eat dinner at 6 pm and don't eat again until breakfast at 7 am, you've fasted for 13 hours.

5. Reduced Caloric Intake: Having an early dinner may reduce the number of calories consumed in a day, as there is less time to eat additional snacks or meals. This can lead to a calorie deficit, which is essential for weight loss.

6. Regulated Hunger Hormones: Eating dinner early can help regulate hunger hormones like ghrelin and leptin, which can influence appetite and the sensation of fullness. This can make it easier to control food intake and avoid overeating.

I have made some tasty recipes for your dinner, which will not only keep you healthy but will give you an amazing inch loss.

1. Mooli ka saag- saute cumin seeds and mustard seeds, with hing and other spices. Add chopped radish greens to it. After 2-3 minutes add chopped radish and salt to it, stir for a while. Cover with a lid and cook for 5-10 minutes. You can garnish it with lemon juice, I personally like this addition but you can skip it as well. Mooli ka saag, or radish greens, is a nutritious leafy vegetable commonly used in Indian cuisine. It offers a range of health benefits, as it is rich in vitamins (A, C, K, B vitamins), minerals (calcium, iron, potassium), and dietary fiber. These nutrients support various aspects of health, including digestive health, bone strength, immune system function, and heart health. Radish greens are also low in calories, making them a valuable addition to weight-conscious diets. Their antioxidant properties, particularly from

vitamin C, protect against oxidative stress and reduce the risk of chronic diseases. Including mooli ka saag in your diet can be a delicious and nutritious way to promote overall well-being.

2. Dry Fruit milk- Soak 5-6 almonds and raisins. Blend it along with skimmed milk, 2-3 dates (after removing their seeds), crushed cardamom and 3 saffron strands. Drink this milk as you like it warm or cold. Women with PCOD and PCOS can replace cow milk with almond milk. Almonds and raisins provide a dose of healthy fats, fiber, and antioxidants, which can aid in controlling appetite and promoting a feeling of fullness. Dates offer natural sweetness and a source of energy without excessive added sugars. Cardamom and saffron add flavor without additional calories. This nutrient-rich beverage can serve as a satisfying and wholesome dinner option, contributing to overall calorie control while providing essential nutrients.

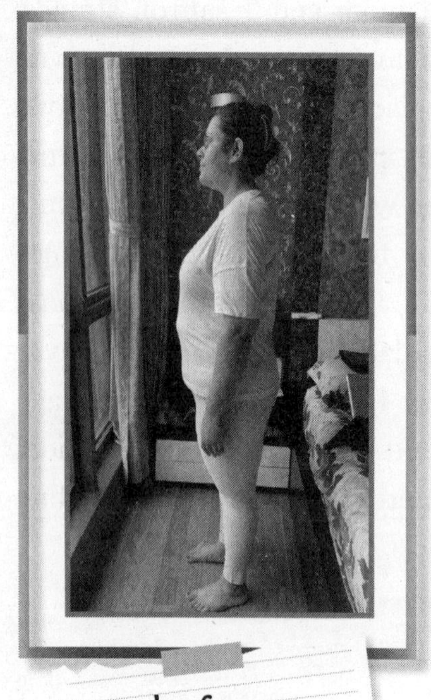

before

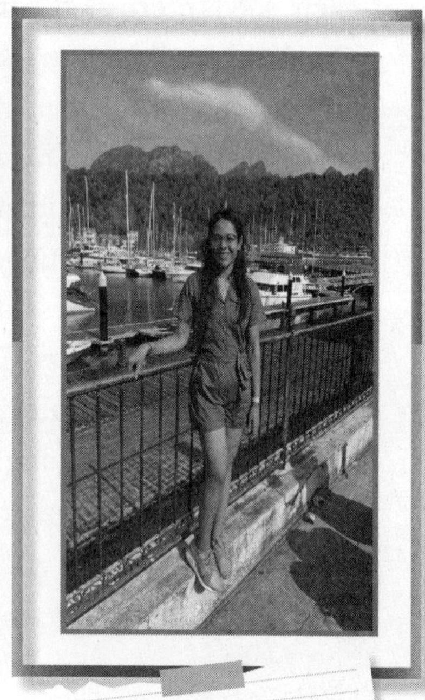

After

Chapter 4

DO YOU KNOW THESE ADDITIONALS OF WEIGHT LOSS?

Diet and lifestyle are two most fundamental and important components of the weight loss equation. And once you get them right, there is nothing that can stop you from losing weight. However, there are certain things that work like additionals in aiding weight loss. This chapter is about these additional methods that you can consider for yourself in addition to the already established fundamentals of this journey.

1. Intermittent fasting-

A fairly popular term and a fairly popular concept of Intermittent fasting recently took over the internet as one of the most effective ways to lose weight. Intermittent fasting is not something that can be attributed to modern times alone. The concept of fasting has been known to our culture and has been a large part of our religious practices as well. However, The modern resurgence of intermittent fasting as a health and weight management strategy happened specifically in 2012, after the BBC2 television Horizon documentary Eat, Fast and Live Longer, where scientific research led by individuals like Dr. Michael Mosley and Dr. Valter Longo reached the masses through television. Dr. Mosley, for example, the popular "5:2 diet," which involves eating normally for any five days and consuming only a very low-calorie intake for the next two non-consecutive days. There are trials and studies going on in various universities and institutes that are more closely studying the effects on intermittent fasting on our bodies. "We have known for almost a hundred years that healthy fasting 1 extends an animal's healthspan and lifespan. Although eating less also slows aging in humans, it can be difficult to follow. Recently, however, studies have shown that intermittent fasting affects aging in a similar way in animals. Since intermittent fasting may be easier to follow than calorie counting, we are excited to see if intermittent fasting may be an easier way to become healthy and slow the aging process," says Dr. Corby Martin, Professor and Director of the Ingestive Behavior, Weight Management and Health Promotion Laboratory at Pennington Biomedical. Fasting is a tricky territory as when you get a solution which has added benefits, we begin to take leverage of it and begin to over exhaust the effectiveness of a solution. Some people think that when intermittent fasting is so effective, I shall not need to regulate my calorie intake and that fasting will take care of everything that I put in my gut. On the contrary fasting is an additional tool that only works when your routines are sorted and when your nutrition is well assimilated in the body. The experts' take on intermittent fasting states, "eat sensibly most of the time, eat nothing for a very small period every now and then and indulge only on occasion. There is research, they claim, to back up the health benefits of sensibly incorporating fasting into your lifestyle."

But if you exploit this tool, it can do more damage than good. If you are conscious of what you eat in the 'eating window', you can lose some really good inches with the help of 'fasting window'. The only type of fasting that I recommend is the Time-restricted eating.

❖ **Time-Restricted Eating:**

- Method: Limiting daily eating to a specific time window, called the 'eating window' and fasting for the remaining time called the 'fasting window'. 16:8, 14:10 , 12:12. For the beginners I suggest you start with a 12:12 diet as it allows you to ease into the process and in the 12 hours of fasting you will mostly be in your sleeping period.
- Who It's Suitable For: Generally, this is suitable for many healthy individuals.

However there are other methods like

❖ **Alternate-Day Fasting**

(Alternating between regular eating days and fasting days which only allow very low-calorie intakes), **5:2 Diet** (Eating normally for five days of the week and for the rest of the two consecutive days consuming only a very low-calorie diet (usually around 500-600 calories), . **Eat-Stop-Eat** (Fasting for a full 24 hours once or twice a week), **Warrior Diet** (Fasting during the day and consuming one large meal in the evening)

But these methods are very harsh on the body that are largely not suitable for those with certain medical conditions, pregnant or breastfeeding women, or individuals with a history of eating disorders. These methods can also cause nutritional deficiencies and can significantly affect your blood-sugar levels.

- This is why I always suggest that for beginners, the best intermittent fasting plan is the 12:12 or to the max 14:10 method as it allows the body to ease into the process as the maximum part of the 12-14 hour fasting window spent sleeping by the individual. One should never go to extremes with these additional tools of weight loss especially with intermittent fasting. The goal should always be in facilitating the body to be healthier and a better version which as a result will help you with a healthier weight.

Moreover there are some people who should never even try intermittent fasting.

These are

1. **Children and Adolescents:** growth and development can be affected in this age group, so it's generally not recommended for individuals under 18 years of age.
2. **Pregnant or Breastfeeding Women:** the mother and the baby during pregnancy require adequate nutrition during this time and fasting can deprive the body of essential nutrients.

3. **Individuals with Eating Disorders:** Those with a history of eating disorders, such as anorexia or bulimia, should avoid intermittent fasting, as it can further complicate unhealthy eating patterns.
4. **People with Certain Medical Conditions:** Individuals with diabetes, hypoglycemia, or other metabolic conditions should never try diet changes or fasting without consulting with a healthcare professional. Fasting can affect blood sugar levels and may require adjustments to medication or dietary plans.
5. **Those on Medications or with Medical Conditions:** Anyone taking medications or undergoing any underlying medical conditions should also consult a healthcare professional before starting intermittent fasting or any diet changes to ensure the safety and efficacy for their particular situation.

My diet plan for intermittent fasting

Let's revise the basics first. The five golden rules that we had discussed before, are to be followed here as well. In the 12 hours period we will take our full meals and for the 12 hour period nothing solid is to be consumed, only liquid is allowed for intake.

Morning tea (7-7:30 AM) - Saunf tea

Breakfast (8-8:30 AM) - Oats paratha

Mid-morning snack (10:00-10:30 AM) - your favorite seasonal and local fruit with 5 soaked almonds

Lunch (1:00-1:30 PM) - protein salad

Evening tea + seeds (4:00-4:30 PM) - Green tea/ Black coffee/ Lemon water with a small bowl of roasted makhana/ roasted chana

Dinner (6:00-6:30 PM) - Soya bowl

Night drink (8:30-9:00 PM) - Jeera tea

For detailed recipes and other food options, you can watch this video about intermittent fasting on my youtube channel. https://www.youtube.com/watch?v=9yU6cu37Y_A&t=383s

2. Detox-

A detox diet plan, often referred to as a detoxification or cleanse diet, is a short-term dietary regimen designed to eliminate toxins from the body and promote overall health and well-being. Proponents of detox diets claim that they can help the body rid itself of harmful substances and support various bodily functions. However, not everyone will tell you that certain detox diets and fasts can even be fatal. Detoxification is one of the natural processes of our bodies. We actually do not need to go to extreme measures to take toxins out of our body because our physical selves have an automatic system setup for that. But this also does not mean that if you keep adding toxins in the form of junk food, alcohol and other harmful substances into your body that it will keep taking it in and there will be no apparent problems rising from it. To this I suggest, the kind of environment we live in and the kind of lifestyle we live, a person can undergo a mild detox regimen every now and then. I also strictly advise that the detox should not go on for more than 2-3 days and 7 days only in special cases as per advised by your nutritionist. The direct goal of detoxification is not to lose weight but to enhance and support our body's ability to function properly so that it can correct problems on its own. Weight loss, here, is not a primary goal but an effect of the process that we follow. During detoxification one should be careful of not exerting their bodies and minds, during this time take plenty of rest and be mindful of the following things.

the key considerations when approaching detox diets:

1. Consult a healthcare professional
2. Understand the purpose
3. Avoid extreme diets
4. Hydrate
5. Choose a well-balanced approach
6. Watch for potential side effects
7. Be aware of weight loss
8. Avoid prolonged detoxes
9. Listen to your body
10. Don't expect miracles
11. Focus on building long-term habits
12. Say no to extreme claims

Most of the detoxes that are suggested by so called experts involve fasting for a prolonged period, or taking only juices or smoothies, or performing self-administered enemas. All these actions fall under the category of extreme measures. Therefore you should always be careful that you only follow the guidelines of registered experts who will not ask you to risk your health and wellbeing for their own benefit. Unfortunately, most detox diets are deficient in protein which negatively affects the body's ability to detoxify because our body needs protein for the enzymatic reactions that are critical to the detoxification process, absence of this does more harm than good.

Fiber is another important nutrient that is found to be lacking in these diets. Fiber helps improve the excretion of toxins through the feces. It can also enhance gut barrier function, which can help protect the organs involved in detoxification from proinflammatory bacteria.

So, if detoxification is so complex and confusing why should one even do it? This is because the studies without a doubt deject the idea of extreme detoxes but it also gives some evidence suggesting that certain, very mild detox measures may also help promote the health of the liver, which is the major site of detoxification, as well as improve the function of enzymes involved in detoxification, given that the measures are well regulated and not harsh on the body.

Detoxification also helps in:

1. **Improved Diet and Eating Habits:** A good and a balanced detox plan encourages participants to eliminate processed foods, added sugars, caffeine, and alcohol, and

instead focus on whole, unprocessed foods like fruits and vegetables. This can lead to better dietary choices and healthier eating habits.

2. **Increased Hydration:** Detox plans often recommend drinking plenty of water, herbal teas, or detox beverages, which can help improve overall hydration and support bodily functions.
3. **Weight Loss:** Some individuals may experience weight loss during a detox plan, particularly if it involves caloric restriction or a reduction in processed foods and empty calories.
4. **Enhanced Energy Levels:** Improved dietary choices and increased hydration can lead to increased energy and vitality for some people.
5. **Better Digestive Health:** Detox plans may promote improved digestive health by encouraging the consumption of fiber-rich foods and reducing processed foods that may be harder to digest.
6. **Mental Clarity:** Some people report increased mental clarity and improved focus during or after a detox plan. This could be due to improved nutrition, better hydration, or a reduction in caffeine intake.
7. **Feeling of Well-being:** Many individuals feel a sense of accomplishment and well-being after completing a detox program, even if the specific detoxification claims are not substantiated by scientific evidence.
8. **Short-Term Reset:** Detox plans can serve as a short-

term reset for individuals who have been following an unhealthy diet or experiencing a period of overindulgence. It can help them return to more balanced eating habits.

And always remember to say 'NO' to the detox plans that are usually very strict and hard on the body. Don't fast for longer periods of days, just relying on smoothies and juices, conducting enemas, as these measures are not safe. Our bodies are very much capable of doing the basic cleaning on its own, we do not need extreme detoxifications. Try basic changes in your food choices, incorporating meals that are cleansing yet nutritious in nature.

3. Exercises:

Exercise is a form of physical activity that is done in order to better one's health or achieve a specific fitness goal. Exercise is often the first advice given to people aiming for weight loss. But exercise alone does not amount to losing those inches. It only works when it is supplemented with a healthy lifestyle and a healthy diet. Once you have built a healthy regimen around that diet & nutrition, you can build a good exercising schedule that will help you to get healthier and get to your perfect weight.

Regular physical activity and exercise offer numerous health benefits, including:

- Improved cardiovascular health, reducing the risk of heart disease and stroke.
- Weight management and body composition improvement.

- Enhanced muscular strength and endurance.
- Better bone health and reduced risk of osteoporosis.
- Improved mental health, including reduced risk of depression and anxiety.
- Increased energy levels and reduced fatigue.
- Better sleep quality.
- Enhanced flexibility and reduced risk of injury.
- Improved balance and coordination.
- Regulation of blood sugar levels, reducing the risk of type 2 diabetes.
- Enhanced immune system function.
- Increased longevity and a reduced risk of chronic diseases.

Given so many benefits of exercising, I always recommend a 30 minute light exercise that suits you well. I am also a believer in exercising what you enjoy. There are some studies done on the link between enjoying a physical activity and its impact on our brain and body. One of the studies stated, "Enjoyment of exercise seems to be a mediator of exercise level. Enjoyment of exercise may be important for the long-term effectiveness of health care-based interventions." Besides exercising what you enjoy, you should also consider these factors while deciding a particular physical activity to include in your daily life.

Choosing the right exercise for weight loss depends on various factors, including your fitness level, preferences, any physical limitations, and the amount of time and effort you're willing to commit. Here are steps to help you choose an exercise for weight loss:

1. **Consult a Healthcare Professional:** it's crucial to consult with a healthcare professional or a registered dietitian before starting any exercise program. The experts with a knowledge of your medical history and any underlying health conditions, can assess the safety and efficacy of a physical activity for your case.
2. **Assess Your Current Fitness Level:** Most people get into heavy exercises without properly assessing their current level of fitness. First you should always determine your current fitness level, as this will help you adjust the intensity and type of exercise that will be appropriate for you. If you're new to exercise or have been sedentary for a while, start with low-impact activities and gradually progress, don't just jump the steps of the process.
3. **Set Clear Goals:** Define your weight loss goals and what you want to achieve with exercise. Do not exercise to just lose weight but do it to improve your overall health and fitness.
4. **Consider Your Preferences:** Choose an exercise that you enjoy and are more likely to stick with in the long run. If you find an activity fun, you're more likely to stay motivated. Consider options like walking, running, cycling, swimming, dancing, or sports you enjoy.
5. **Track Your Progress:** Keep a record of your workouts,

including the type, duration, and intensity of exercise and the response of your body to it. This can help you stay motivated, informed and provide you with data to make necessary adjustments to your routine.

6. **Stay Hydrated and Eat Balanced:** With exercise comes the importance of hydration. Proper hydration is essential, and it's vital to maintain a balanced support to your weight loss efforts. Exercise alone is not enough.
7. **Listen to Your Body:** Pay attention to your body and any signs of fatigue or pain, don't ignore your body's call for help. While some fatigue and exertion is good, overexertion or pushing too hard can lead to injuries and setbacks. Rest when needed and allow your body to recover.
8. **Seek Support:** Consider working with a personal trainer or joining a fitness class or support group to stay motivated and receive guidance.

4. Protein rich diet-

Protein is required for building and sustaining all our bodily processes. Right from a cell to our whole body, everything is fundamentally made up of protein. Our muscles are made up of proteins and when there is a deficiency of Protein during the weight loss process, it disturbs the bodily processes reducing the substance of muscle mass also called as the lean body mass. Maintaining lean body mass/muscle mass is essential for sustaining a healthy metabolic rate, preserving strength and function, and keeping a healthy body composition. When you lose muscle mass, your basal metabolic rate (BMR) can decrease, making it more challenging to maintain or continue to lose weight. Reduced muscle mass also results in decreased physical strength and functional capacity, impacting your ability to perform daily activities and exercise effectively.

To mitigate protein loss during weight loss and promote a healthy lean body mass, you should focus on a few key strategies. First and foremost, ensure your protein intake is adequate to your specific body-weight-height requirements. Also check with your health care provider if there are any specific changes required to suit your medical history. Protein requirements can vary, but a general guideline is to aim for about 0.8-1.2 grams of protein per kilogram of body weight per day. However, individual needs may differ, so it's best to consult with a registered dietitian for personalized recommendations.

Incorporate regular exercise into your fitness routine. Physical activity stimulates muscle growth and preservation, even while losing weight. While exercising aim for a holistic work out plan and work to engage all major muscle groups without stressing out your body. A gradual weight loss approach is also recommended, as slow and steady weight loss is more likely to preserve lean body mass than rapid weight loss.

As I always say, diet is the most important component of our health, so ensure you're getting essential macro and micronutrients through whatever you are eating. Additionally, staying well-hydrated is important for muscle function, as dehydration can contribute to muscle cramps and fatigue. Rest and recovery are equally important, as they allow your muscles to repair and grow. Get enough sleep and avoid overtraining. These steps combined together will help you to maintain a healthy lean body mass and preserve your muscle mass.

If you find it challenging to strike the right balance between weight loss and muscle mass maintenance, consider working with a certified dietitian or a fitness trainer who can help you create a personalized plan that supports your weight loss goals while preserving lean body mass. Ultimately, remember that achieving a healthy and sustainable weight loss is not just about losing weight but about optimizing your long-term well-being and overall health. I always tell my clients to never keep weight loss as their main goal because this goal can drive them towards taking extreme measures which will only end in disappointment. Whereas if your focus is on bettering your overall health, you will never ever try or do anything which you know can end up harming you. Moreover when we work with a holistic health approach, weight loss happens as the most obvious result.

Protein plays a significant role in weight loss and weight management due to several key mechanisms and benefits. Here's how protein helps in weight loss:

- **Satiety and Appetite Control:** Protein helps you feel full and satisfied after a meal. Therefore it is a highly satiating nutrient. It triggers the release of hormones that sends a signal to your brain if you've had enough to eat. As a result, it stops you from overeating, leading to a reduction in overall calorie intake.

- **Calorie Burning:** The thermic effect of food (TEF) is a term referring to the energy expenditure required to digest, absorb, and metabolize the nutrients present in your diet. Protein has a higher TEF compared to carbohydrates and fats, which means your body requires you to burn more calories to process and use protein for energy. Thus, protein intake in itself helps with calorie budget regulation.
- **Muscle Preservation:** When you're on a calorie-restricted diet for weight loss, your body may break down both fat and muscle for energy. Consuming an adequate amount of protein can help preserve lean muscle mass, which is important for maintaining metabolic rate and overall strength. More muscle means a higher basal metabolic rate (BMR), which can help you burn more calories even at rest.
- **Stabilizing Blood Sugar Levels:** Protein-rich meals help with a gradual release of glucose into the bloodstream. This happens because protein can slow down the digestion and absorption of carbohydrates, leading to a more stabilized absorption and circulation system. This helps prevent spikes and crashes in blood sugar levels and as a result reduces cravings.
- **Cravings Reduction:** High-protein diets are satiating in nature and studies have shown them to reduce

cravings for unhealthy, high-calorie foods. This can make it easier for people on their weight loss journeys to stick to a healthy eating plan and avoid overindulging in processed and sugary foods.

You can either maintain a good protein intake by a diet enriched with protein or you can take naturally easily available foods like **sattu powder**. Protein is one of the most essential macronutrients for our body and it is equally essentially for our weight loss. Most people do not pay much attention to protein intake which stops them from effectively losing weight. Thus you have a protein rich diet while working for your weight loss or include such natural options like sattu powder in your diet to balance any nutritional deficiencies in your food.

For a detailed protein rich diet plan, you can watch this video on my youtube channel.

Benefits of sattu powder-

- **Rich in Protein:** rich source of amino acids, making it a good protein option for vegetarians and vegans.
- **High in Fiber:** rich in dietary fiber, aids in digestion, promote regular bowel movements, and helps prevent constipation.
- **Low in Fat:** low in fat, making it a suitable choice for those looking to reduce their fat intake.
- **Rich in Nutrients:** contains essential vitamins and minerals, including B vitamins, calcium, magnesium, and iron, contributing to overall health and well-being.

- **Energy Booster:** quick and sustained source of energy due to its carbohydrate content. It can be especially useful for athletes and individuals with active lifestyles.
- **Hydrating Properties:** Has a cooling and hydrating effect. It helps prevent dehydration.
- **Weight Management:** The combination of protein and fiber in sattu can help with weight management by promoting satiety and reducing overall calorie intake.
- **Digestive Health:** The fiber in sattu aids in promoting a healthy gut and can contribute to improved digestive health.
- **Blood Sugar Control:** low glycemic index, meaning it doesn't cause rapid spikes in blood sugar levels. It can be a good addition to the diet for those with diabetes.
- **Versatility:** Sattu can be consumed in various forms, such as as a drink, paratha (flatbread), or mixed with yogurt. Its versatility allows for different culinary applications.
- **Gluten-Free Option:** If made from chickpeas or other gluten-free grains, sattu can be a suitable option for those with gluten sensitivities or celiac disease.
- **Economical and Homemade:** Making Sattu powder at home is a cost-effective way to ensure the quality and purity of the product. You can avoid additives or preservatives that might be present in store-bought versions.

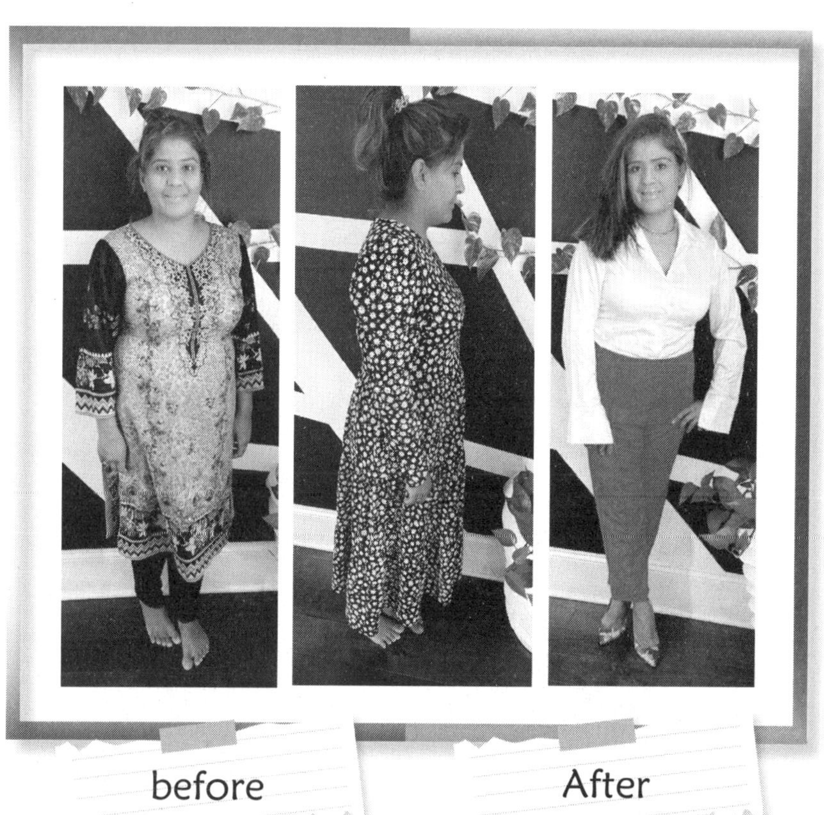
before
After

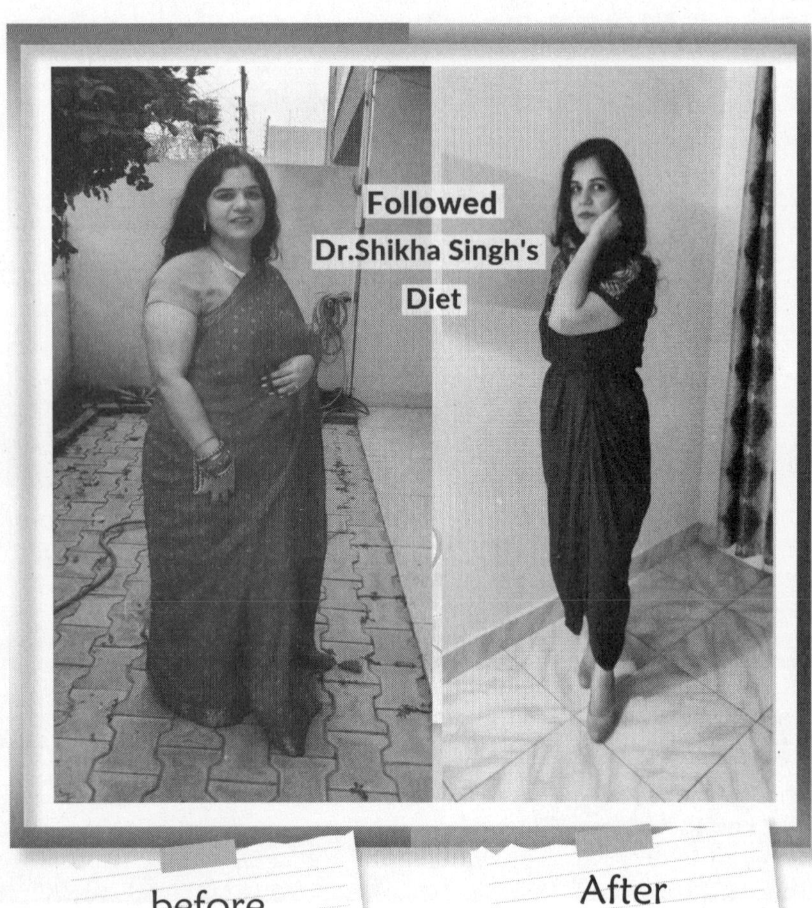
Followed
Dr.Shikha Singh's
Diet
before
After

Chapter 5

CAN I LOSE WEIGHT IF I HAVE?

- PCOD/PCOS
- Thyroid
- Diabetes
- High cholesterol

PCOS/PCOD-

Polycystic ovary syndrome (PCOS), is a condition where the ovaries, a female reproductive organ, are unable to complete the process of ovulation. Female bodies have a pair of ovaries in their lower abdomen. These ovaries produce an egg every month which when fertilized leads to pregnancy and otherwise the process ends up as menstruation. In PCOD/ PCOS the body suffers with hormonal imbalance and the female hormones like LSH, estrogen, progesterone are not synthesized to the required quantity because they are replaced by male hormones, androgen, testosterone etc. The hormonal imbalances disrupt the normal process of ovulation, leading to irregular or absent ovulation (release and maturation of a female egg). WHen there is no formation and maturation of eggs, there is no reason for the body to undergo menstruation or prepare for pregnancy. PCOD/PCOS occurs in a person in the reproductive age between 15-44 years. In today's times around 20% of the female population is suffering from PCOD/PCOS. It is characterized by a range of signs and symptoms related to hormonal imbalances and disruptions in the normal functioning of the ovaries. While the terms PCOS and PCOD are often used interchangeably, PCOS is the more commonly used term.

Some symptoms of PCOS include:

- **Irregular Menstrual Periods:** Irregular, infrequent, or absent menstrual periods.
- **Ovarian Cysts:** small, fluid-filled sacs or cysts, which are often detected during ultrasound examinations.
- **Excess Androgen Production:** Elevated levels of male hormones cause symptoms like acne, excessive hair growth esp. Facial hair, hair loss & male-pattern baldness, snoring.
- **Insulin Resistance:** Many individuals with PCOS/PCOD have insulin resistance, which causes higher sugar levels in the bloodstream. This can also increase the risk of type 2 diabetes.
- **Weight Gain:** Weight gain and obesity are common symptoms of PCOS. Weight is both a cause and a symptom of PCOD/PCOS.
- **Skin Issues:** Acne and the development of dark patches

on the neck and in body folds.

- **Fertility Issues:** Irregular ovulation and hormonal imbalances can make it challenging to conceive. PCOS is one of the leading causes of infertility in women.
- **Mood Disorders:** mood disturbances, such as depression and anxiety.

What Causes PCOS/PCOD?

- **Genetics:** There is evidence to suggest a genetic component to PCOS. If you have a family history of PCOS, you may have a higher risk of developing the condition.
- **Hormonal Imbalances:** various reasons like poor diet and lifestyle can lead to hormonal imbalances. These imbalances cause elevated levels of androgens (male hormones) such as testosterone and suppress levels of female hormones like estrogen and progesterone in the body. These hormonal imbalances cause a number of symptoms including weight gain and irregular or absent ovulation.
- **Insulin Resistance:** Some individuals with PCOS develop insulin resistance, which means their cells do not respond efficiently to a hormone called insulin. Our pancreas produces a hormone called insulin. Whenever we eat anything it releases glucose in our body. Insulin takes care of using this glucose and assimilating it in the cells. In simple terms, insulin pushes the glucose into the cells so that the cells can convert it into energy. However when we eat excess sugar than required, the glucose keeps circulating in the bloodstream without proper assimilation,

this signals our body to produce more insulin which slowly moves towards the case of insulin resistance. Moreover higher levels of insulin in turn causes the body to increase the synthesis of male hormones called androgens and decreases the synthesis of female hormones. Therefore a female body fails to function properly in terms of what it normally does.

- **Inflammation:** Chronic low-grade inflammation causes hormones to go haywire. This sets the cycle for hormonal imbalances which in turn increase the levels of male hormones in the body while suppressing the levels of female hormones. Inflammation also contributes to insulin resistance and affects ovarian function.
- **Lifestyle Factors:** Obesity is often associated with PCOS. Excess body fat, particularly around the abdomen, can exacerbate insulin resistance and hormonal imbalances. Additionally, sedentary lifestyles and poor dietary choices may contribute to the development and progression of PCOS.
- **Environmental Factors:** Some environmental factors, such as exposure to endocrine-disrupting chemicals, have been suggested as potential contributors to the development of PCOS, although more research is needed in this area.

Here are certain dietary factors that may play a role in the progression of PCOS/PCOD:

Highly Processed and Sugary Foods, Saturated and Trans Fats, Excessive Caffeine, Dairy Products, Alcohol, High

Glycemic Index (GI) Foods, Caffeine

Treatment of PCOD/PCOS

Normally the patients with PCOD/PCOS are treated with medicines which suppress the levels of male hormones in your body and increase the production of female hormones. This process treats the symptoms and you can then see that the menstruation cycle returns to its normality. However, this treatment is only made to suppress the symptoms, it doesn't cure anything at its root. There is nothing that your body is doing on its own, it's working with the aid of medicines that are doing what your body is supposed to do naturally. This is the reason why, when you stop taking your medicines, you find yourself back at square one. Remember when I told you, "when your diet is wrong, medicine is of no use and when your diet is right, medicine is of no need." This saying applies here as well. The first thing to do is always correct your lifestyle and diet. Because the benefits of a right diet and lifestyle can overshadow the impact of bad genes, hormonal imbalances, environmental factors and can also correct other underlying conditions that are aggravating your problem. Along with the diet and lifestyle I always stress on the importance of creating a holistic approach towards your health and wellbeing.

Dealing with PCOD/PCOS can be challenging. But if you begin to take control of certain factors, you'll see your body will take control of the rest by itself. Lifestyle can be improved by following the 5 golden rules that I have discussed in detail in the second chapter.

- Sleep on time
- Drink 3-3.5 liters of water everyday
- Do a mild Exercise everyday for half an hour
- Monitor your weight every morning
- Manage stress

Now since we have revised the 5 golden rules, let's start with the Diet plan that I generally recommend to my clients suffering from PCOD/PCOS.

Foremostly, there are things that you should Completely cut off from your diet because they are extremely harmful for a person suffering from PCOD/PCOS.

These are

❖ **Sugars & refined carbohydrates:** Foods that are high in refined carbohydrates and sugar can cause rapid spikes in blood sugar levels, which as we discussed above, causes PCOD/PCOS symptoms to exacerbate . eg. white bread, sugary cereals, pastries, and sugary snacks, Soda, fruit juices, and other sugary drinks.

❖ **Dairy Products:** Some individuals with PCOS may be sensitive to dairy products and moreover dairy products cause inflammation in the body. Consider reducing or eliminating dairy and replacing it with dairy alternatives like almond or soy milk.

❖ **Processed Foods:** contain unhealthy fats, sugars, and additives. These can contribute to weight gain and insulin resistance, which are common concerns in PCOS.

Diet plan:

1. **Morning drink-** Turmeric tea
2. **Breakfast-** Masala idli/Weight loss chicken sandwich/ masala oats/jowar chilla
3. **Mid-morning meal-** any local and seasonal fruit; suggestive- 1 Pomegranate /1 bowl of mixed berries (if it's available)
4. **Lunch-** Oats mango smoothie/other oats smoothies/1 bowl of daal/Moong dal chaat/Moong dal chilla
5. **Evening snack-** Tomato smoothie/ 1tbsp mixed seeds
6. **Dinner-** Ragi soup// grilled chicken/grilled fish/3 eggs recipes/ salad
7. **Night drink-Cinnamon tea**

You can check out the detailed recipes and other food options on my youtube channel.

Benefits of these ingredients

❖ **Turmeric:**

- Turmeric contains curcumin, which has anti-inflammatory and antioxidant properties.
- It may help reduce inflammation and improve insulin sensitivity, which can be beneficial for PCOS.

❖ **Rawa (Semolina):**

- Rawa is a whole wheat product that is a good source of complex carbohydrates.

- It can provide sustained energy and help stabilize blood sugar levels when consumed in moderation.

❖ **Oats:**

- Oats are a good source of fiber, particularly beta-glucans, which can help regulate blood sugar and improve insulin sensitivity.
- They may also aid in weight management, which is important for PCOS.

❖ **Chicken:**

- Lean sources of protein like chicken can be part of a balanced diet for managing weight and supporting hormone balance in PCOS.

❖ **Jowar (Sorghum):**

- Jowar is a whole grain rich in fiber and nutrients.
- It can help with blood sugar regulation and weight management.

❖ **Berries:**

- Berries are low in sugar and high in antioxidants and fiber.
- They can help control blood sugar levels and reduce inflammation.

❖ **Mango:**

- Mango is a fruit that is moderately high in natural sugars. While it's nutritious, it should be consumed in moderation to manage blood sugar levels.

❖ **Moong Dal (Green Gram):**

- Moong dal is a good source of plant-based protein and fiber.
- It can support satiety and blood sugar regulation.

❖ **Tomato:**

- Tomatoes are low in calories and rich in antioxidants, including lycopene.
- They can help reduce inflammation and improve overall health.

❖ **Ragi (Finger Millet):**

- Ragi is a whole grain rich in fiber and essential nutrients.
- It can help stabilize blood sugar levels and contribute to a balanced diet.

❖ **Fish:**

- Fatty fish like salmon and mackerel are excellent sources of omega-3 fatty acids, which have anti-inflammatory properties and may improve insulin sensitivity.

❖ **Eggs:**

- Eggs are a good source of high-quality protein and various nutrients.
- They can help with satiety and hormone balance.

❖ **Salad:**

- Salads made with a variety of vegetables are low in calories and high in fiber, vitamins, and minerals.

- They can support weight management and overall health.

❖ **Cinnamon:**

- Cinnamon may help improve insulin sensitivity and lower blood sugar levels.
- It can be a beneficial spice for people with PCOS.

2. Thyroid -

What is Thyroid?

Thyroid is a butterfly-shaped gland situated in your throat. It is an important part of the endocrine system, it is responsible for producing and releasing hormones like T3 and T4 that play a vital role in regulating various bodily functions, including metabolism, energy production, and overall health.

Thyroid hormones influence functions like metabolism, Temperature Regulation, Heart Rate, Digestion, Growth and Development.

Sudden onset of symptoms like gaining weight, tiredness, low energy, sensitivity to cold temperatures, constipation, dry skin, irregular periods, infertility and cholesterol problems, can signal hypothyroidism.

Our bodies are capable of fighting diseases and infections by producing antibodies in the body. But sometimes this immune reaction attacks the body's own cells causing the occurrence of diseases. This similar thing causes some patients to develop hypothyroidism, where the body's immunity starts attacking thyroid cells, causing this gland to become underactive or overactive.

What happens when the thyroid gland becomes dysfunctional?

When the thyroid gland becomes dysfunctional and does not produce or regulate thyroid hormones properly, it can lead to a range of health problems. The two main types of thyroid dysfunction are hyperthyroidism and hypothyroidism. We will mainly deal with hypothyroidism here, as this is the type which causes weight gain in patients.

Hypothyroidism:

- Hypothyroidism is a condition in which the thyroid gland does not produce enough thyroid hormones, leading to a slowed metabolism.
- The most common cause of hypothyroidism is autoimmune thyroiditis (Hashimoto's disease), which results in gradual destruction of thyroid tissue. Other causes can include thyroid surgery, radiation therapy, or certain medications.
- Symptoms of hypothyroidism can include:
    - Fatigue
    - Weight gain
    - Cold intolerance
    - Dry skin and hair
    - Constipation
    - Depression

- Muscle weakness
- Joint pain

- Hypothyroidism can affect various bodily functions and, if left untreated, can lead to complications like goiter (enlarged thyroid gland), heart problems, and myxedema coma (a life-threatening condition). Treatment usually involves lifelong thyroid hormone replacement therapy with medications like levothyroxine. However, on the other hand, I am living proof of the fact that there is a more natural way of treating hypothyroidism and that it can be corrected with a good lifestyle and dietary improvements.

Causes of Hypothyroidism:

- **Autoimmune Thyroiditis (Hashimoto's Disease):** This is the most common cause of hypothyroidism. It occurs when the body's immune system mistakenly attacks and damages the thyroid gland, leading to a gradual decrease in thyroid hormone production.
- **Iodine Deficiency:** Insufficient iodine in the diet can lead to hypothyroidism, as iodine is a key component of thyroid hormones. This cause is fairly common in some regions in India where iodized salt is not routinely used.

  Other causes are more towards the genetic and surgical implications side which can damage the thyroid gland and lead to hypothyroidism.

  Some medications can also interfere with thyroid function and cause hypothyroidism.

Lastly, conditions affecting the pituitary gland or hypothalamus can disrupt the release of thyroid-stimulating hormone (TSH) and, consequently, thyroid hormone production (central hypothyroidism), causing hypothyroidism.

Weight loss for thyroid patients

The most visible symptom of hypothyroidism is weight gain. Patients with this problem find it almost impossible to lose their extra weight, which causes immense demotivation and also adds to many health risks. There are many reasons why hypothyroidism causes weight gain as a symptom. But primarily, the problem lies with the inability of our body to burn calories. See, normally when we are at rest there is a certain portion of our energy that goes into supporting our involuntary life functions like breathing, circulation etc. These activities continue even at rest thus they require our bodies to burn a certain amount of calories. However, with patients that have a dysfunctional thyroid, their bodies slow down the fundamental processes of life, therefore requiring relatively less calories to be burnt even at rest, as compared to other individuals. This is why people with hypothyroidism often suffer from weight gain problems. Besides this a lot of lifestyle changes both cause and result from hypothyroidism like, Slowed Metabolism, Reduced Energy Expenditure, Increased Fat Accumulation (Hypothyroidism can lead to changes in the way your body stores and uses fat), Fluid Retention, Changes in Appetite and Eating Habits (increased food cravings or overeating), fatigue, low energy levels, and muscle weakness causing reduction in physical activity, insulin sensitivity and Hormonal imbalance (affects leptin and ghrelin causing appetite and energy imbalance). These causes and effects make it extremely difficult for patients with dysfunctional thyroids to lose and regulate their weight.

I too weighed 110 kilos and one of the major reasons behind this number was hypothyroidism. If, being a Thyroid patient I could lose around 50 kilos with some lifestyle and dietary changes, you too can do it. And I challenge you to get up and do this task which I know seems impossible to you.

Losing weight can be beneficial for individuals with thyroid disorders, particularly those with hypothyroidism or Hashimoto's disease, as it can help improve thyroid function and overall health. Here are some ways in which weight loss can have a positive impact on the thyroid:

- **Improved Insulin Sensitivity:** Weight loss can enhance insulin sensitivity, making it easier for the body to use glucose for energy. In cases where insulin resistance is present, improved insulin sensitivity can help stabilize blood sugar levels and reduce the risk of developing type 2 diabetes, which is more common in individuals with thyroid disorders.
- **Enhanced Hormone Regulation:** Weight loss can help regulate hormones in the body, including thyroid hormones. In some cases, losing excess weight can alleviate the strain on the thyroid gland and potentially reduce the required dosage of thyroid

hormone replacement medication for individuals with hypothyroidism.

- **Lower Inflammation:** Excess weight can lead to chronic inflammation, which may contribute to thyroid dysfunction. Weight loss can reduce inflammation, potentially easing the strain on the thyroid gland and improving its function.
- **Improved Metabolism:** Shedding excess weight can lead to an increase in metabolic rate, which can help with energy levels and overall vitality. This can be particularly important for individuals with hypothyroidism who often experience fatigue and a slowed metabolism.
- **Cardiovascular Health:** Maintaining a healthy weight can reduce the risk of cardiovascular diseases, such as heart disease and high blood pressure, which are more prevalent in individuals with thyroid disorders.
- **Reduced Symptom Severity:** Weight loss can alleviate some of the symptoms associated with thyroid disorders, such as joint pain, fatigue, and mood disturbances.
- **Support for Autoimmune Conditions:** In the case of autoimmune thyroid conditions like Hashimoto's disease, weight loss can help manage the autoimmune response and inflammation, potentially reducing the severity of the condition.

Things to avoid

1. Cauliflower
2. Broccoli

3. Spinach
4. Coffee
5. Soya chunks
6. Gluten

Things to include

1. Selenium rich foods like eggs, whole green gram, brown rice, Quinoa
2. Curd
3. Pumpkin seeds
4. Nuts esp. Brazil nuts (avoid peanuts)
5. Flax seeds
6. Dairy Products

So we are going to lay some ground rules here, because there are certain parts of the routines that you should never miss.

But before this you remember the 5 golden rules that I told you about in the last chapters? They apply here as well.

So,

- Sleep on time
- Drink 3-3.5 liters of water everyday
- Do a mild Exercise everyday for half an hour
- Monitor your weight every morning
- Manage stress

Starting with your daily routine, the first thing you should do in the morning is take your thyroid medicine and then do the rest of the things like use the washroom. After this drink some water and then take a gap of 45 minutes before taking any other liquid or food.

Diet Plan

45 minutes after taking your medicine-

take **Morning drink** - apple cider vinegar in lukewarm water

After a gap of 30 minutes- take your Breakfast- Brown Rice/Vegetable Quinoa/ Besan Chilla/Kuttu chilla/Moong dal chilla and replace your tea/coffee with a small bowl of dahi without salt

Lunch- Beans/ tinda/ Pumpkin/Chia pudding/smoothies

Evening tea- Green tea + 5 almonds +2 walnuts+ 1 tbsp pumpkin seeds

Dinner- The most important thing to consider here is that you need to have your dinner before 8PM in the evening. If you have dinner after 8 PM, all your efforts even combined together will also not amount to any weight loss.

Eggs/ Thandai/ Turmeric Milk/ Boiled or roasted Chicken breasts

Avoid salt in your dinner, instead use black pepper and lemon juice.

Night Drink- Coriander seed Tea

You can check out the detailed recipes and other meal options on my Youtube channel.

3. Diabetes -

A lot of people presume that since their parents are diabetic, there is a 100% necessity that they too will develop diabetes accruing it to their genes. However, diabetes is a lifestyle disorder, it occurs due to irresponsible dietary makeup and lifestyle errors that slowly and gradually amount to this condition. Then why is it that a lot of people actually acquire diabetes, seeming like it is a disease flowing from their family tree? This is because when a family lives together, their food habits and lifestyle are similar. These changes cause people to develop similar kinds of lifestyle disorders including diabetes, high cholesterol, hypothyroidism etc. Although we cannot completely negate the role of bad genes, we can actually say that a good diet and a healthy lifestyle can definitely overshadow the impact of genetic makeup in our bodies. If these are certain things that follow a larger part of your life, there are chances that you might develop diabetes in the future.

Now I want you to pay attention to the details I am going to uncover here. This is the science behind the occurrence of diabetes in the human body. As we all know, when we eat or drink anything, our body converts that input into glucose and then energy. However in patients with diabetes, this mechanism of conversion of food into energy, begins to falter. There is an organ in our body called the pancreas and it is responsible for producing a hormone called insulin. Whenever we eat anything it releases glucose in our body. Insulin takes care of using this glucose and assimilating it into the cells. In simple terms, insulin pushes the glucose into the cells so that they can convert it into energy. However in diabetic patients, the insulin is unable in pushing glucose into the cells causing it to circulate in the bloodstream without proper assimilation. This is the reason why our blood tests would record a higher level of blood-sugar in the body. Since there is no conversion of glucose into energy happening inside the body, you will often find diabetic patients to experience increased fatigue and tiredness. This need for energy causes for them to experience symptoms like

- **Polyphagia (Increased hunger):** When your body's cells are not getting the energy they need due to insufficient insulin or insulin resistance, you may feel hungry more often.
- **Polydipsia(Increased thirst):** High blood sugar levels can cause dehydration, leading to increased thirst.
- **Unexplained Weight Loss:** People with diabetes, especially type 1 diabetes, may experience unexplained weight loss even though they are eating more to compensate for increased hunger. However on the flip side there can also be diabetes related weight gain. Diabetes itself does not directly cause weight gain, but the management and treatment of diabetes can sometimes lead to weight changes.
- **Polyurea(Frequent Urination):** Excessive thirst and increased urination are common early signs of diabetes. When blood sugar levels are high, the kidneys try to remove the excess sugar by excreting it through urine.

- **Ketoacidosis:** It occurs when the body doesn't have enough insulin to process sugar for energy. Instead, it starts breaking down fat for energy, which produces chemicals called ketones. Ketones can build up in the blood, making it too acidic.
- **Fatigue:** Diabetes can lead to a lack of energy and persistent fatigue, as the body's cells are not effectively utilizing glucose for energy.
- **Blurred Vision:** High blood sugar levels can affect the shape of the lens in your eye, leading to temporary vision changes.
- **Slow Wound Healing:** The body in diabetes breaks down protein to create energy for the body. Thus, the actual function of protein is replaced for producing energy for the body, hampering the body's ability to repair itself, leading to slow healing of cuts, sores, and bruises.
- **Frequent Infections:** People with diabetes may be more susceptible to infections, especially urinary tract and yeast infections.
- **Tingling or Numbness:** Nerve damage (diabetic neuropathy) can cause tingling or numbness in the hands or feet.
- **Dry Skin and Itching:** Diabetes can lead to dry skin and itchiness, often as a result of poor circulation and damaged nerves.

Types of Diabetes:

- **Insulin-Dependent Diabetes (Type 1 Diabetes):** In this type of diabetes, the body loses the ability to synthesize insulin as the body's own immune system begins to mistakenly attack the insulin-making cells in the pancreas. Since there's no insulin being made, people with type 1 diabetes have to be administered insulin either through injections or an insulin pump. In this condition, the body's own natural mechanism to produce insulin gets hampered thus it requires insulin from outside to maintain normal functioning. In most cases, type 1 diabetes is diagnosed in patients before the age of 30, with a peak incidence in childhood and adolescence.
- **Non-Insulin-Dependent Diabetes (Type 2 Diabetes):** Type 2 diabetes is different. From type 1 diabetes, as here the body's own ability to make insulin is not hampered but insulin's ability to function effectively takes a hit. In this type, the body still makes insulin, but it doesn't work as well as it should. In type 2 diabetes, the insulin receptors present on our cells, fail to recognize insulin, causing the assimilation of glucose to falter in its mechanism.
- It can also be related to insulin-resistance that the body develops as a result of other disorders. It's like having keys to open doors, but the locks default in allowing a key to open the door. Consider this example, imagine that there is a house and there is a main door to this house which is guarded by a watchman. Every person

who enters the house goes through a check by this watchman. Now equate this house with your body and this watchman guards whatever goes inside the cells. The watchman recognizes insulin very well and allows anyone that comes along with insulin inside of the house. However, in diabetes, this watchman sort of forgets the appearance of insulin and loses familiarity with it. And whoever comes along with insulin is no longer allowed to get inside of the cells. This is exactly what happens to the glucose that comes along with insulin at the membranes of our cells. Thus the glucose keeps running in the bloodstream, amounting to the higher blood-sugar levels.

I always say that in order to treat any disease you should first correct your diet and lifestyle. To begin with, here are a few things that you should avoid and a few things that you should include in your diet to correct the diabetic condition. And later in this section I will share a diet plan with you that you can follow to lose weight that comes as a result of diabetes.

Avoid

1. Processed food
2. Refined flour
3. Refined sugar

Include

1. Diet changes

2. Exercise
3. medication

A word of caution that I always put out for my diabetic patients is to never try any random diet plan that you discover without the help of an expert. The major complication with diabetes is that if your blood sugar level drops uncontrollably with a particular change that you inculcate in your life, it can lead to a situation of hypoglycemia (dangerously low blood sugar level in the body). This condition is far more dangerous than hyperglycemia and can even be fatal. Therefore it is always advisable to consult with your doctor or your health provider to ensure the safety of a diet plan for you.

I am a certified nutritionist and a doctor, so whatever i am going to tell you next, you can follow these suggestions without any worry. These suggestions are beneficial to your body and are written after taking diabetes as a medical condition into consideration. Here are my 5 golden rules to begin your lifestyle changes with.

❖ **Regular Physical Activity:**

- Engage in regular exercise, which can help lower blood sugar levels and improve insulin sensitivity.
- Aim for at least 30 minutes of mild intensity activity every day, or exercise with an activity that you enjoy the most. You can also try light yoga and pranayam. The point initially, is to get your body moving without straining it a lot.

❖ **Stress Management:**

- Chronic stress can raise blood sugar levels. Practicing stress reduction techniques, such as mindfulness, yoga, or meditation, can help manage stress.

❖ **Adequate Sleep:**

- Aim for 7-8 hours of quality sleep per night, meaning going to bed around 10:00 PM and getting early around 6:00 AM. As we have already discussed, the timings of your sleeping schedule matter a lot as only deep sleep happening at the right time frame, results in positive health impacts. Otherwise, no matter how much you sleep, if it's not at the right time, it will do more harm than good.

❖ **Regular Monitoring:**

- Monitor blood glucose levels as advised by your healthcare provider to track your progress and make necessary adjustments to your lifestyle.

❖ **Drink 3-3.5 liters of water everyday:**

- Hydration is one of the most important parts of a healthy lifestyle.

Diet plan:

- Consume food in every 2 hours and never skip your meal
- Morning drink (7:00-7:30 AM): Methi tea
- Breakfast (8:00-8:30 AM): Amaranth roti + 1 small bowl karele ki sabzi + 1 small bowl salad

- Mid-Morning breakfast (10:00-10:30 AM): 1 bowl jamun / 1 bowl papaya /1 bowl apple (whichever is locally and seasonally available)
- Lunch (1:00-2:00 PM): Stuffed paratha + 1 small bowl of salad
- Evening snack (4:00-4:30 PM): chana chaat salad with sprinkled flax seeds
- Dinner (7:00-8:00 PM): Multigrain roti + 1 bowl sabzi + 1 bowl salad
- Night drink (9:00-10:00 PM) : Turmeric milk

Individuals with diabetes who are looking to lose weight should focus on a balanced diet that helps manage blood sugar levels and supports weight management. Here are the potential benefits of the foods mentioned above for people with diabetes aiming to lose weight:

- **Methi (Fenugreek):** lower blood sugar levels and improve insulin sensitivity due to their high fiber content.
- **Amaranth:** high in fiber and protein, which can help control blood sugar and promote a feeling of fullness, aiding weight management.
- **Karela (Bitter Gourd):** lower blood sugar levels and may support weight loss due to its low calorie and carbohydrate content.
- **Salad:** low-calorie and high-fiber option that can help control appetite and assist in weight management.

- **Jamun (Indian Blackberry):** blood sugar-lowering effect, low-calorie fruit option.
- **Papaya:** low-glycemic fruit, rich in vitamins and fiber.
- **Apple:** High in fiber, regulates blood sugar levels, controls appetite.
- **Chana (Chickpeas):** High in protein and fiber, stabilizes blood sugar levels and promotes fullness.
- **Flax Seeds:** High in fiber and healthy fats, manages blood sugar and promotes a feeling of fullness.
- **Multigrains:** Source of complex carbohydrates, fiber, and nutrients for a balanced diet.
- **Turmeric Milk:** anti-inflammatory properties and improves insulin sensitivity.

4. Cholesterol-

Cholesterol is a waxy, fat-like substance that is used as a building block in the body. Now, you might be wondering that I said the same thing about proteins as well. Protein and cholesterol, even though both are associated with building and repairing the body, there are differences in the way they conduct this function. Think of protein as the workers in a construction crew. They are the building blocks that help construct and repair things in your body, similar to how the construction workers perform their job. Proteins as we had discussed before are essential for the various tasks that occur in our body. From making cells to organs to muscles to enzymes and to helping your body function correctly, proteins are like the most essential ingredients our body uses. Now, picture cholesterol as the drivers of a car that transport the building materials required for the construction and repair to occur. Cholesterol doesn't build or repair things directly, but it plays an important role in transportation of nutrients and maintaining your body's functions. There are two types of drivers:

- **Low-Density Lipoprotein (LDL):** These drivers are a bit like "bad" drivers who tend to speed and cause traffic accidents. They transport cholesterol to different parts of your body. If there are too many of them, they can create traffic jams (cholesterol buildup) in your arteries, leading to problems like heart disease.
- **High-Density Lipoprotein (HDL):** HDL drivers, on the other hand, are like responsible, safe drivers. They help clean up the highway by picking up the "bad" drivers (LDL) and taking them back to the garage (your liver) to be fixed or removed.

Cholesterol is essential for our bodies thus it is abundantly present in the natural diets we take. Additionally cholesterol is also synthesized within our bodies indicating that it is an essential to the functioning of our system. Here are some primary sources of cholesterol:

❖ **Dietary Sources:**

- Animal Products: Common sources include red meat, poultry, fish, and dairy products like milk, cheese, and eggs. Organ meats, like liver, contain particularly high amounts of cholesterol.

- Shellfish: Certain types of seafood, such as shrimp, lobster, and crab, contain relatively high cholesterol levels.
- Processed and Fried Foods: Some processed and fast foods, like hamburgers, fried chicken, and processed baked goods, can contain high levels of unhealthy trans fats, which can raise your LDL (bad) cholesterol.

❖ **Endogenous (Internal) Sources:**

- Your liver produces cholesterol naturally. Even if you don't consume cholesterol through your diet, your body will still make it because it's essential for various bodily functions.

High-Density Lipoprotein (HDL) is like a superhero for your body. HDL which is the good cholesterol works like a little cleaning crew in your bloodstream. It goes around picking up the "bad" cholesterol (Low-Density Lipoprotein or LDL) that's causing trouble in your arteries and takes it to the liver where it gets broken down. LDL is referred to as "bad" cholesterol because it can clog up your arteries, causing cardiovascular diseases and other serious health conditions. When your arteries are clear and open, it's easier for your heart to pump blood and oxygen to your body. This means your heart doesn't have to work as hard, reducing the risk of heart problems.HDL makes sure of this by carrying the "bad" cholesterol away which clears the arteries of any blockage.

Since we have established that HDL is 'good cholesterol' and LDL is' bad cholesterol, we shall now discuss the reasons for high levels of LDL, its complications and the corrective measures for it.

What causes high levels of LDL?

❖ **Dietary Choices:**

- Consuming a diet high in saturated and trans fats, found in red meat, full-fat dairy products, fried and processed foods, and baked goods, can raise LDL cholesterol levels.

❖ **Lack of Physical Activity:**

- A sedentary lifestyle with little or no physical activity can contribute to higher LDL cholesterol levels.

❖ **Obesity:**

- Excess body weight, particularly when it's concentrated around the abdomen, is often associated with elevated LDL cholesterol.

❖ **Genetics:**

- Some individuals have a genetic predisposition to high LDL cholesterol, a condition known as familial hypercholesterolemia. In such cases, the body has difficulty regulating cholesterol levels, leading to elevated LDL cholesterol from a young age.

❖ **Certain Medical Conditions:**

- Conditions such as diabetes, hypothyroidism, and kidney disease can lead to higher LDL cholesterol levels.

❖ **Smoking:**

- Smoking damages blood vessels and can lower levels of HDL (good) cholesterol, which, in turn, may lead to increased LDL cholesterol.

❖ **Age and Gender:**

- Cholesterol levels tend to increase with age. Men typically have higher LDL cholesterol levels than premenopausal women, although women's levels may rise after menopause.

❖ **Medications:**

- Some medications, including certain antipsychotic drugs and corticosteroids, can increase LDL cholesterol levels.

❖ **Dietary Cholesterol:**

- While dietary cholesterol has a smaller impact on blood cholesterol levels compared to saturated and trans fats, consuming excessive amounts of dietary cholesterol, like that found in egg yolks and organ meats, can contribute to higher LDL cholesterol in some people.

As I always say, any disease can be remedied with lifestyle and dietary changes, here is what I particularly suggest for patients suffering from high levels of bad cholesterol.

Keeping the basics same, lifestyle shall be corrected with my five golden rules which are,

- **Eat Right:** well-balanced diet and portion sizes.

- **Regular Exercise:** Choose activities that you enjoy to make exercise a sustainable part of your lifestyle. Exercise what you enjoy for 30 minutes everyday.
- **Adequate Rest and Sleep:** 7-8 hours of quality sleep every night. Sleep around 10 PM and wake up around 6:00 - 6:30 AM.
- **Manage Stress:** Manage stress to avoid hormonal dysfunction
- **Stay Hydrated:** Drink 3-4 liters of water everyday. Proper hydration is essential for various bodily functions.

Along with lifestyle changes, this is the diet plan that you can follow to keep your cholesterol levels regulated.

This Diet plan will help you reverse your high LDL levels, weight loss and improve your overall health.

- Morning drink (7:00-7:30 AM): Turmeric tea
- Breakfast (7:00-7:30 AM): Oats paratha + 1 small bowl low fat curd (If you want to take tea or coffee, please avoid sugar, jaggery or any other sweetener, although you can use 1-2 stevia leaves)
- Mid-Morning breakfast (10:00-10:30 AM): any locally and seasonally available fruit (preferably apple or strawberry) + 5 soaked almonds
- Lunch (1:00-1:30 PM): Oats smoothie + 1 full bowl salad (without salt)

- Evening snack (4:00-5:00 PM): 1 small bowl Oats chivda + green tea/lemon water
- Dinner (6:00-7:00 PM): 1 big bowl Masala bhindi + 1 bowl salad
- Night drink (9:00-10:00 PM) : Flax seeds water

Find more meal options and detailed recipes on my channel on youtube.

❖ **Turmeric:**

Curcumin in turmeric has antioxidant and anti-inflammatory properties, which can contribute to reducing inflammation and oxidative stress related to high LDL cholesterol.

❖ **Oats:**

Oats are high in soluble fiber, which can help lower LDL cholesterol levels by binding to cholesterol and preventing its absorption in the gut.

❖ **Almonds:**

Almonds are a source of healthy monounsaturated fats, which can help reduce LDL cholesterol.

They also contain fiber and antioxidants that support heart health.

❖ **Strawberry:**

Strawberries are rich in antioxidants, including anthocyanins and vitamin C, which can help reduce oxidative stress and inflammation linked to high LDL cholesterol.

❖ **Apple:**

Apples are high in soluble fiber, particularly pectin, which can help lower LDL cholesterol levels by reducing cholesterol absorption.

❖ **Salad:**

Salads made with a variety of fresh vegetables are typically low in saturated fats and calories, making them a heart-healthy choice.

The fiber in salads can help lower LDL cholesterol and promote overall heart health.

❖ **Bhindi (Okra):**

Okra is rich in soluble fiber, which can help lower LDL cholesterol levels.

It can also improve digestive health, which can indirectly affect cholesterol absorption.

❖ **Flax Seeds:**

Flax seeds are an excellent source of soluble fiber and omega-3 fatty acids, both of which can help reduce LDL cholesterol levels.

The fiber in flax seeds binds to cholesterol, preventing its absorption.

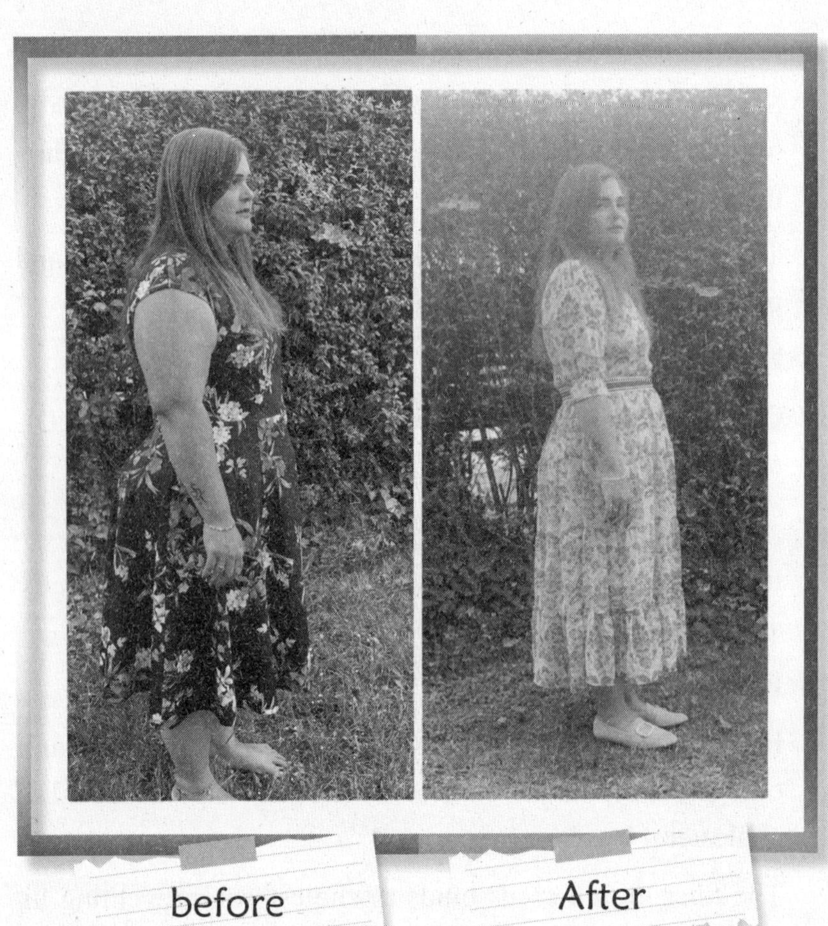
before
After

Chapter 6

DIET PLAN FOR TEENAGERS

I understand how heartbreaking it is to see your body undergoing changes which are out of your control.Teenage can be a daunting time, all of a sudden your face is full of acne, body hair begin to grow, you undergo periods for the first time and there is a range of new moods and feelings that you begin to feel. This is what teen age is mostly related to. However in the last 15 years, there has been another factor that is becoming highly attached with teenagers and that is the problem of obesity and being overweight. An observational study done on a total of 385 adolescents of district Rohtak, Haryana showed that there is a prevalence of a total 19.3% of childhood overweight and obesity in India. Experts at NCBI says, "The ongoing pandemic of obesity, particularly, that of childhood obesity has emerged as a huge challenge for epidemiologists, program managers, and policy makers around the world. The economic implications of childhood obesity will be huge." But not getting into the bigger repercussions of this pandemic, I want to bring this issue to its cause, so that we can in the most gentle way understand and treat what is just a symptom of the range of things that are going wrong for this generation.

Teenage years are one of the most stressful periods in a child's life. The pressure of examinations, competitions, securing a good college, entrance examinations, peer pressure, changing bodies all adds to what already is a chaotic time. These times are confusing for a child who is transitioning into an adult life as there is so much to learn, explore, adjust to and change with. To this there is also an added pressure that is emerging for teenagers these days and this is the pressure of being overweight and obese. If I revisit my teenage self, I too remember comparing myself to the image of the "popular girls" who were lean and fit. I on the other hand was overweight weighing 110 kilos and the stress of this, added to my life as a student and a young teenage girl. With my education in medicine and then nutrition, I discovered a full proof solution to my obesity and lost around 50-55 kilos naturally. Today, I wish I had an understanding of obesity back then so I would have not tortured myself with trying different random things just to get the weight off me. However, my dear reader, if you are a teenager reading this, you do not have to worry. I understand the stress and pressure you are going through in this age and I am here to ease away your troubles by simple mantras and a tasty diet plan that you will at least never worry about your weight again.

What is the major mistake that you might be making as a teenager that has caused your weight gain?

Teenage is scientifically referred to as adolescence, it is a period of one's life falling between 12-18 years of age. Teenage is a crucial period of our lives as during this period a lot of growth and changes occur in our body. These changes and growth prepare us to gradually enter into adulthood. Since this age is determined by physical and mental development, it's without a doubt that the body would require a healthy diet rich in calories and protein to make up energy for these activities, during this time. However, teenagers usually fulfill their requirements for this extra energy by eating empty calories they get, by binging on junk food. This puts the body into stress and most of the time these empty calories become the major reason for obesity in teenagers. There's also a growing trend among teengers where the majority of them are going to bed late at night. This habit owes its credit to the heavy burden of studies for some and that late-at-night habit to binge watch content on the internet for others. In addition, the very nature of a modern student life creates constant cravings which are again satiated by unhealthy snacks like 2 minute noodles, chips, biscuits etc. I understand that you guys have a lot on your plate. There is a mountain of syllabus to be completed, never ending tests and extra co-curriculars. With so much going on, it is hard for you to pay attention to your health. Most teenagers, I can bet, don't have proper breakfast, often skip their meals, are glued to computer and phone screens, and don't even leave their seats for most part of their days. But one thing that you should understand is your actions today will loop your body into survival mode forever and hamper your body-mind from experiencing proper growth and development..But then "karein kya?" I understand that the world of health ,diet and nutrition is so confusing. There is so much information out there, especially for young kids like you that it is almost impossible to come up with a single line of action that is actually good for you. This is why I am going to lay down simple steps that you can do in order to get back to a healthy lifestyle and lose the extra inches as a natural result. I don't want you to stress out on the do's and don'ts of weight loss. All I want from you is an open mind that is here to understand, learn, unlearn and implement. In this chapter you will get everything that you will ever need to end your confusion around your changing body and weight gain.

Other factors that cause teens to become overweight?

The following are some of the factors that may contribute to overweight adolescents:

- Easy availability of food, especially high-calorie snack food
- Parents' attitudes toward food
- Eating more fast foods
- Using food as a reward or punishment to change behaviors
- Lack of exercise
- TV watching and snacking
- Not knowing how to eat healthy
- Similar patterns of lifestyle and diet to parents' and family members' that are overweight

Teenagers have specific nutritional needs because they are going through a period of rapid growth and development. It's essential for teenagers to consume a well-balanced diet that provides them with the necessary nutrients for optimal growth, cognitive development, and overall health. Some of the key nutrients that are essential for teenagers include:

- **Protein:** Protein is crucial for growth and repair of body tissues, especially during adolescence when growth spurts occur. Good sources of protein include lean meats, poultry, fish, beans, legumes, dairy products, and tofu.
- **Calcium:** Calcium is essential for building and maintaining strong bones and teeth. Teenagers need an adequate intake of calcium to support their growing bones. Dairy products, fortified plant-based milk, leafy green vegetables, and fortified cereals are good sources of calcium. Around 800 mg daily requirement.
- **Iron:** Iron is necessary for the formation of red blood cells and carrying oxygen throughout the body. Adolescents, especially girls, are at risk of iron deficiency due to increased blood volume during puberty. Good sources of iron include lean red meat, poultry, fish, beans, lentils, and fortified cereals.
- **Vitamin D:** Vitamin D is important for calcium absorption and bone health. It can be obtained from sunlight exposure and dietary sources like fortified dairy products, fatty fish, and supplements if necessary.
- **Fiber:** Fiber is essential for digestive health and helps

prevent constipation. It can be found in whole grains, fruits, vegetables, and legumes.

❖ **Folate (Vitamin B9):** Folate is important for cell division and DNA synthesis. It is found in green leafy vegetables, legumes, and fortified cereals.

❖ **Omega-3 fatty acids:** Omega-3 fatty acids, particularly DHA and EPA, are important for brain development and cognitive function. Fatty fish like salmon, mackerel, and flaxseeds are good sources.

❖ **Vitamin A:** Vitamin A is important for vision, skin health, and immune function. It can be found in sweet potatoes, carrots, and dark leafy greens.

❖ **Vitamin C:** Vitamin C is important for skin health and the immune system. It is found in citrus fruits, strawberries, and bell peppers.

❖ **Vitamin E:** Vitamin E is an antioxidant that helps protect cells from damage. Nuts, seeds, and vegetable oils are good sources.

❖ **B vitamins:** B vitamins, including B6, B12, and riboflavin, are essential for energy production, red blood cell formation, and overall growth and development. They can be found in a variety of foods, including meats, dairy products, and fortified cereals.

❖ **Magnesium:** Magnesium is important for muscle and nerve function, as well as bone health. It can be obtained from foods like nuts, seeds, whole grains, and leafy green vegetables.

- **Potassium:** Potassium is necessary for maintaining proper muscle and nerve function, as well as regulating blood pressure. It is found in foods like bananas, oranges, and potatoes.

Things to avoid

1. Say no to packaged food esp. with preservatives, sugar and salt
2. I wouldn't recommend fasting for teenagers as it robs their body off essential nutrients that are required during this time.
3. Going to bed late
4. Binging on junk food

I always say this, the fact that you have listened to the things that i have to say, is never enough. Understanding is only the first step towards achieving your goal. The next step is to learn, unlearn and then build your actions into a consistent habit. See, the thing is, if you are thirsty and I tell you that there is a glass of water on the table nearby. You have received the information and the solution, and to the maximum I can get that glass for you but until and unless you yourself drink the water from that glass your thirst will never be quenched. Similar to this, you are eager to lose weight and I am here to tell you science backed information and solutions that you can learn in order to achieve your goal. But until and unless you follow knowledge with implementation, nothing is going to change. So, whatever you learn please practice and implement it, don't just shelve it for later use.

Now, let's begin with the real talk. Whenever I suggest a diet plan to someone, I tell them the importance of lifestyle as well. See, lifestyle and diet go hand in hand. One without the other is of no use. Before, you begin to bring dietary changes in your life. You should first begin to understand what it means to have a healthy lifestyle and build one. In almost all the previous chapters I have mentioned my 5 golden rules. These rules revolve around sleep, mental health, consistency, hydration and exercise. These are five golden areas that if you correct as part of your lifestyle, you will see amazing results not just in terms of weight loss but also in terms of your overall health.

5 golden rules

1. Getting 7-8 hours of sleep at the right time (10:00PM-6:00AM)

Examinations often come with the immense challenge of first completing our syllabus, then doing revisions and then practicing for the finale. Children respond to this by squeezing their sleep time to accommodate the extra study hours required for preparation. This results in a combination of negative behaviors like going to bed late and waking up late in the morning or going to bed late and waking up early or avoiding sleep altogether for a long stretch. However, these actions do more harm than good. Staying up late is relatively easier than waking up early so most students choose the first option. However this simple negligence causes a lot of troubles for your body and mind. There is a gland in our body called adrenal, and it produces hormones like cortisol and adrenaline. These hormones have their own set of functions to perform but when their levels in the body increase, it creates a fight or flight system in the body. Your brain gradually loses its capacity for optimum functioning, similarly the body loses out on energy and undergoes a myriad of hormonal disturbances. When you don't get enough sleep, your body produces more of a hormone called ghrelin, which makes you feel hungry. It also reduces the production of another hormone called leptin, which tells your brain that you're full. So, when you're sleep-deprived, you tend to feel hungrier and end up eating more. Lack of sleep can make you crave unhealthy, high-calorie, and sugary foods. You're more likely to reach for snacks and junk food when you're tired, which can lead to weight gain.When you're tired, you have less energy for physical activity and exercise. This can make it harder to burn calories and lose weight because you might not feel like being active. Poor sleep can slow down your metabolism, which is how your body burns calories. A slower metabolism means you burn fewer calories, making it more challenging to lose weight.

2. Drink 3-3.5 liters of water everyday.

You see, water is like a magical elixir for our bodies. It helps us in so many ways, and one of those ways is by supporting weight loss. Drinking plenty of water helps control your appetite, supports your metabolism, and helps you burn more calories. It also keeps your body functioning at its best, which is essential for successful weight loss. Just remember to sip on water throughout the day, and you'll be doing a big favor for your health and your weight loss journey.

If you have difficulty keeping up with a hydration schedule, you can work around digital alarms that keep you adhered to a routine with constant reminders.

3. Exercise-

Think of your body like a car. When you exercise, it's like driving the car around. The more you drive (exercise), the more fuel (calories) you use up.

So, regular exercise is like taking your car for a spin to use up the extra fuel in your tank. If you rev up the engine, you for sure are using up high amounts of fuel but you are also causing wear and tear to the engine. Additionally speeding up the process also brings with it the potential hazards of safety against accidents and damage. This is why I never suggest you indulge in intensive exercises. However I also don't suggest you sit idle, glued to a couch all day. Both are extremes of a situation thus you should always choose a middle path. In this case the middle path is for you to be active and moving all day, doing pranayam or light yoga, or exercising what you enjoy. Play a sport that you really enjoy for half an hour a day and that should do you good.

4. No stress-

Picture your body's metabolism as a hose carrying water. Stress is like a knot in the hose. It restricts the flow of progress (calories burnt), making it harder for your metabolism to work efficiently. When you manage stress, it's like unknotting the hose, allowing the water (calories) to flow freely. In yet another example Imagine your body is like a car on a journey to a healthier weight. Stress acts like a big roadblock on your weight loss journey. It's like pressing the brakes on your car when you want to go forward. When you're stressed, your body releases hormones that can make you eat more, especially unhealthy stuff, and it can slow down your metabolism, making it harder to lose weight. So, avoiding stress is like removing that roadblock or taking your foot off the brakes, allowing you to move forward smoothly on your weight loss journey. When the road is clear, it's much easier to make healthy choices and shed those extra pounds.

So, managing stress is a crucial part of your weight loss plan! There is a portion of stress that I understand is inevitable and it comes to us as part and parcel of life. However, a lot of stress acts as a demotivator and a causative factor of a lot of lifestyle diseases. So learn to manage and respond healthily to stressful events in life.

5. Regular monitoring-

Think of your weight like a savings account. When you check it regularly, it's like keeping an eye on your money. If you see any changes, it's easier to notice and manage them early. Monitoring your weight daily can help you stay aware of how your choices, like food and exercise, are affecting your weight. What kind of changes in your weight is a particular action, bringing. Keep a journal and plot a bigger picture of your weight loss journey. With this habit you're more likely to stay on track and make adjustments if needed. If you notice any unusual changes, you can address them sooner, making it easier to reach your weight loss goals. However, remember that your weight can naturally fluctuate from day to day, it's just one part of your health journey, not the whole story. So, don't stress out but use this as a method to paint an objective representation of your weight loss.

Disclaimer- Each individual body requires nutrients based on his/her own height, mass, etc. However there is a general plan that I am giving out here. For further clarifications and a detailed diet plan as per your own needs, you can always consult your healthcare provider or a certified nutritionist. If there are any underlying health conditions, then it becomes of utmost necessity that any dietary changes that you plan on incorporating, you first consult with your doctor who has the knowledge of your particular case.

Diet plan for teenagers who wish to lose weight naturally without compromising on their growth and nutritional requirements.

- Morning Drink- lemon drink
- Breakfast-peanut butter banana sandwich
- Mid-morning snack- Fruit chaat
- Lunch- Weight loss brown rice + 1 small bowl curd +1 large bowl salad
- Evening snack- mint shikanji + 1 small bowl roasted chana/makhana

- Dinner - Moong dal dosa + homemade chutney
- NIght drink- Jeera tea (for 15 days) / lukewarm water(for 15 days)

Here are the benefits of these foods for teenagers looking to lose weight:

- **Peanut butter:** Good source of protein and healthy fats, aiding satiety.
- **Banana:** Provides fiber and natural sweetness, a healthy snack choice.
- **Lemon:** Supports digestion and adds flavor to water without calories.
- **Moong dal (green gram):** High in protein and fiber, promoting fullness.
- **Chana (chickpeas):** Rich in protein, aiding in appetite control.
- **Brown rice:** Offers complex carbohydrates for sustained energy.
- **Curd (yogurt):** High in protein, probiotics for gut health.
- **Salad and vegetables:** Low in calories, high in nutrients, filling and healthy.
- **Shikanji (lemonade):** A low-calorie beverage to replace sugary drinks.
- **Fruits:** Provide fiber, vitamins, and natural sugars for energy.

- **Jeera (cumin seeds):** May help digestion and reduce bloating when used in cooking.

You can also find other food options and detailed recipes that are equally benefiting and exciting, on my youtube channel.

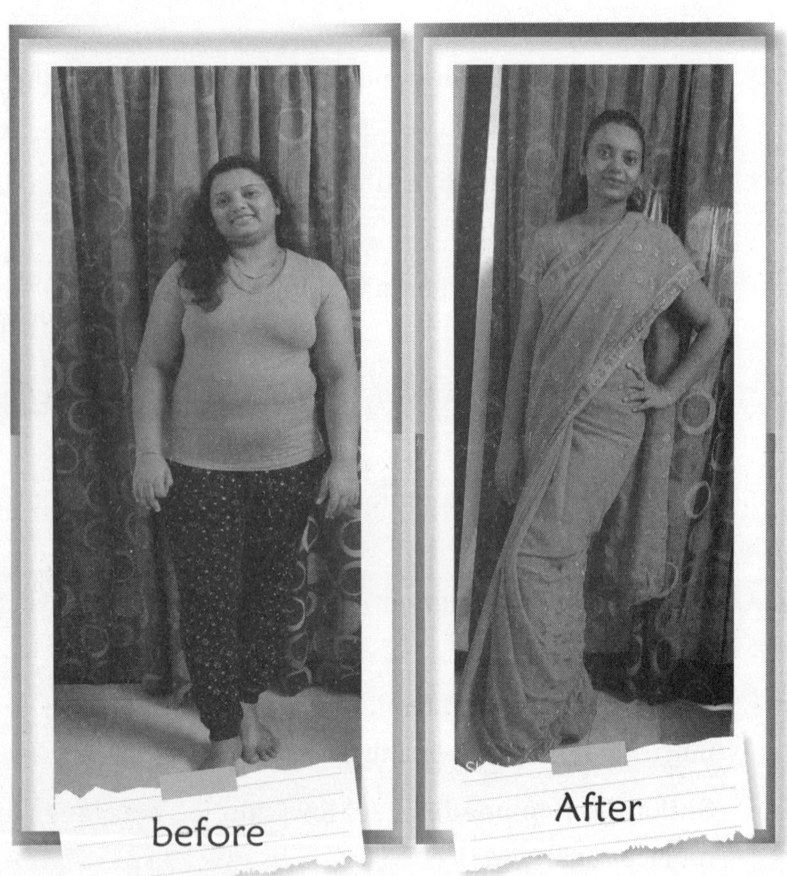

Chapter 7

A CHAPTER DEDICATED TO MY WOMEN READERS!

These are statements from a research study, "The multinomial analysis found that women aged 35 years and above are 5 times more likely to be overweight and 12 times more likely to be obese than women of 15-24 years. Many studies have attempted to determine the causes behind this association between overweight or obesity and demographic covariates. Among all, physical activity declines, along with metabolic rate, in the middle years of women. On the other hand, the energy requirement decreases; therefore, even regular or routine eating may lead to weight gain." In another study done during the COVID-19 pandemic, it was found that "The implications of even modest weight gain at a population level in women could translate into more diabetes, heart disease, cancers and other serious obesity-related health problems over the coming decades in these populations unless action is taken to reverse the effects of lockdown."

Recent studies have found that women are more perceptible to weight gain than men. This can be accrued to the rising cases of PCOD/PCOS, hypothyroidism, Vitamin and other nutritional deficiencies, sedentary lifestyle for office women, pregnancy related weight gain and most importantly stress. In this chapter we are going to look into two monumental phases that a woman goes through, menstruation and pregnancy. Both these natural processes for a majority of women have been disrupted owing to the rapidly changing environment, unhealthy food and lifestyle. Irregular, painful and uncomfortable periods have both emerged as a cause and effect of obesity for young women. And the alarming rise in cases of infertility and obesity in women speaks volumes of all the things that are going wrong in the female body and mind. Let's first start with menstruation.

1. Periods- A lot of my clients find themselves confused with the question, as to what is the process of weight loss during menstruation. Do we continue the same diet, same routine during this time? I will try to answer all such questions in this section.

   To begin with, whenever I discuss a weight loss strategy centered around a health issue, my approach and my solution for it are always two pronged. I always try to give you an approach that targets both weight loss as well as the root cause of that health condition. Similarly my solution also builds on two aspects; that is lifestyle and diet. For menstruation too, my approach is not just to give you a go ahead for exercising and following a diet on your periods but to give you a solution that keeps you on your journey to weight loss without harming your body or depriving it of essential nutrients. I don't ever advise you to starve or exercise intensely during your usual days and I would never ever ask you to do these things during menstruation. A lot of my clients who are dealing with obesity or are overweight, also face problems during their period cycle. They experience a range of symptoms called menstrual symptoms that make it difficult for them to function normally during these days. However I have also seen cases where menstrual symptoms had no connection with obesity but these occurrences were comparatively fewer than the ones that actually showed a connection between the two. See the thing is, both obesity/overweight and menstrual symptoms are linked to poor lifestyle and dietary choices. Since our plates and our schedules comprise more unhealthy food and unhealthy practices, the prevalence of painful or uncomfortable periods is on the rise.This is a statement from a published research study, "Obesity in adolescence is also associated with greater menstrual cycle irregularity and the polycystic ovary syndrome (PCOS), which can result in infrequent or absent menstrual periods, and heavy menstrual bleeding." A Preliminary analysis by Harvard school, reveals that there are a wide range of menstrual cycle symptoms. Out of the first 10,000 participants who enrolled and 6,141 participants who tracked their period symptoms, data was collected to understand the nature of menstrual symptoms. Study found that the most commonly tracked symptom was abdominal cramps, which was reported by

83% of the participants. Bloating was the second most reported symptom (63% of participants), and tiredness was the third (61% of participants). But are painful and uncomfortable periods normal?

According to Ayurveda, painful and uncomfortable periods are a result of an imbalance in the two doshas, particularly Vata and Pitta doshas. The specific symptoms and the underlying causes of discomfort can vary from person to person. However it has been understood that Vata and pitta dosha create these problems during menstruation-:

- **Vata Imbalance:** Painful periods are often attributed to an excess of the Vata dosha, which is associated with qualities like dryness, coldness, and instability. Vata imbalances can lead to symptoms such as irregular periods, abdominal cramps, and heightened sensitivity to pain.
- **Pitta Imbalance:** Excessive heat or imbalanced Pitta dosha may result in heavy bleeding, inflammation, and irritability during menstruation. Women with a Pitta imbalance may experience more intense symptoms.

Ayurvedic treatments for menstrual discomfort typically aim to balance the doshas. They may include dietary changes, herbal remedies, lifestyle modifications, and practices like yoga and meditation.

Research has shown a clear link between obesity or being overweight and various aspects of the menstrual cycle.

- Irregular Menstrual Cycles

- Amenorrhea(absent periods)
- Heavy or Prolonged Menstrual Bleeding
- Polycystic Ovary Syndrome (PCOS)
- Fertility Issues
- Increased Risk of Endometrial Cancer

What is menstruation?

Every month the female body prepares for an entire cycle which it anticipates might lead to fertilization of the egg and creation of a human life. Synthesis of the female egg occurs in the ovaries and it matures every month descending to the uterus for fertilization and then implantation. The body prepares for this by thickening the uterus lining and making it all ready. However, when the egg is not met by a successful fertilization, the uterus lining breaks down signaling the body to restart the process once again. This is a monthly cycle in the female body and the shedding of the uterus is what causes the bleeding in menstruation.

What disrupts this cycle?

The menstrual cycle is a complex and delicate process that can be influenced by various factors. Disruptions in the menstrual cycle can occur for a variety of reasons, including:

❖ **Hormonal Imbalances:**

- Polycystic Ovary Syndrome (PCOS): PCOS is a common hormonal disorder that can lead to irregular or absent periods due to elevated levels of androgens (male hormones).

- Thyroid Disorders: Hypothyroidism (underactive thyroid) and hyperthyroidism (overactive thyroid) can affect the production of hormones that regulate the menstrual cycle.
- Premature Ovarian Insufficiency (POI): POI, also known as early menopause, can cause irregular periods or amenorrhea due to decreased ovarian function.

❖ **Weight Fluctuations:**

- Obesity: Excess body weight can lead to hormonal imbalances, irregular periods, and an increased risk of conditions like PCOS.
- Underweight: Being significantly underweight or having an eating disorder can disrupt the menstrual cycle, causing amenorrhea or infrequent periods.

❖ **Medications and Birth Control:**

- Some medications, such as certain antipsychotics, antidepressants, and hormonal contraceptives, can impact the menstrual cycle.
- Birth control methods like hormonal IUDs or implants can alter menstrual bleeding patterns.

❖ **Medical Conditions:**

- Conditions like endometriosis, uterine fibroids, and adenomyosis can cause heavy, painful periods and irregular bleeding.

- Chronic illnesses, such as diabetes, can affect hormone regulation and menstrual regularity.

❖ **Excessive Exercise:**

- Overtraining or intense exercise can lead to a condition known as exercise-induced amenorrhea, where periods may stop due to low body fat and energy availability.

❖ **Sudden Changes:**

- Rapid weight loss, sudden dietary changes, or significant lifestyle changes can disrupt the menstrual cycle.

❖ **Perimenopause and Menopause:**

- As women approach perimenopause (the transition to menopause), menstrual cycles can become irregular and eventually stop altogether.

❖ **Smoking and Alcohol:**

- Smoking and excessive alcohol consumption can disrupt the menstrual cycle and increase the risk of fertility problems.

What are menstrual symptoms?

These symptoms can vary from person to person in terms of severity and type. Some common menstrual symptoms include:

- **Abdominal Cramps:** Menstrual cramps, also known as dysmenorrhea, are a common symptom. Abdominal cramps occur due to the contractions of the uterine muscles when the uterine wall begins to shed. These cramps can range in intensity from mild to severe and may also be accompanied by lower back pain.

- **Breast Tenderness:** Breast tenderness and swelling can occur in many individuals due to hormonal changes, particularly estrogen, during menstruation.
- **Mood Swings:** Mood swings can occur due to hormonal fluctuations that can affect mood and emotions, leaving an individual with feelings of irritability, sadness, anxiety, or even anger.
- **Fatigue:** Menstruation can cause some people to feel more tired than usual during their cycle.
- **Bloating:** water retention and abdominal bloating can occur due to hormonal fluctuations during menstruation. It can also be linked to changes in metabolism during this time.
- **Headaches:** Some individuals suffer from headaches, including those of the intensity of migraines, in the days leading up to menstruation.
- **Food Cravings:** A lot of people get cravings for quick calories especially those types of food that are often high in sugar, salt, or fat.
- **Nausea:** Nausea can be a less common symptom but it has been reported by some people as a symptom of PMS.
- **Digestive Issues:** Changes in hormone levels can lead to digestive symptoms like diarrhea or constipation.

- **Acne and Skin Changes:** Hormonal fluctuations can also affect the skin, potentially leading to acne breakouts or changes in skin texture.
- **Sleep Disturbances:** Some individuals experience difficulty in getting enough sleep or getting a good quality sleep during their cycle. Some also experience changes in their sleep patterns during their menstrual cycle.
- The role of diet and lifestyle is huge in the occurrence of menstrual symptoms. For example, menstrual cramps are often caused by the release of natural chemicals called prostaglandins, these chemicals cause the uterine muscles to contract more forcefully leading to severe cramps and discomfort.
- Fluctuations in hormones, primarily estrogen and progesterone, play a significant role in the menstrual cycle. These hormonal changes can contribute to various symptoms, including mood swings, breast tenderness, and bloating.

A good diet can play a role in helping to regulate prostaglandins and estrogen, two important hormones involved in the menstrual cycle. While diet alone may not completely control these hormones, it can contribute to maintaining a more balanced hormonal environment. Here's how a good diet can influence prostaglandins and estrogen:

❖ **Prostaglandins:**

- Prostaglandins are natural chemicals that are

responsible for conducting some essential functions in the body. These vital functions include regulation of inflammation, blood flow, and uterine contractions during menstruation. As we discussed, when the egg is not fertilized, the whole preparations that a female reproductive system makes, including the thickening of uterus lining, begins to break down. Prostaglandins play a big role in creating contractions that help shed the uterus lining. However, when the levels of prostaglandins are higher, it causes the contractions to increase in severity and intensity resulting in painful cramps.

Consuming Foods rich in omega-3 fatty acids, such as fatty fish (e.g., salmon, mackerel), flaxseeds, chia seeds, and walnuts, can help reduce the production of inflammatory prostaglandins. These fatty acids have anti-inflammatory properties and may alleviate menstrual pain and discomfort.

❖ **Estrogen:**

- Estrogen is a group of hormones that helps regulate the menstrual cycle by coordinating the timing of ovulation and the buildup of the uterine lining. Certain lifestyle choices and poor nutrition can cause these levels to decrease below normal. Low levels of estrogen cause a lot of problems for the body, making it difficult for menstruation to occur properly and can also cause problems in pregnancy.

Foods like soy products, flaxseeds, and whole grains contain phytoestrogens(plant estrogen) that may help balance estrogen levels by either mimicking the effects of natural estrogen. This can be particularly helpful for women experiencing estrogen imbalances, such as those with menstrual symptoms.

❖ **Stress:**

- is also a factor that contributes to the discomfort experienced during menstruation. In previous chapters we have established how cortisol and adrenaline affect our body. So, I will not repeat it again. However a good diet and lifestyle can help regulate these primary hormones involved in the cycle and target both overweight and menstrual symptoms.

Regulating your menstrual cycles requires a combined improvement in diet as well as your lifestyle. Once again let's revise the 5 golden rules that have been created to build a healthy lifestyle in the most easy and natural way for you .

5 golden rules to a healthy lifestyle

1. Regular Physical Activity:

- Although you should engage in a mild intensity exercise regularly for the other days of the month, during menstruation you can keep your exercise really simple and easy on the body. Aim for a 30 minutes pranayam or very light yoga. The point is to listen to your body and not put a lot of strain on yourself during this period.

2. Stress Management:

- Chronic stress can disturb hormones. So, practicing

stress reduction techniques, such as mindfulness, yoga, or meditation, can help manage stress.

3. Adequate Sleep:

- Aim for 7-8 hours of quality sleep per night, meaning going to bed around 10:00 PM and getting early around 6:00 AM. As we have already discussed, the timings of your sleeping schedule matter a lot as only deep sleep happening at the right time frame, results in positive health impacts. Otherwise, no matter how much you sleep, if it's not at the right time, it will do more harm than good.

4. Regular Monitoring:

- Monitor your weight every morning and track your progress to make necessary adjustments in case you need them.

5. Drink 3-3.5 liters of water everyday:

- Hydration is one of the most important parts of a healthy lifestyle.

I am always asked for diet and lifestyle solutions that not only help with weight loss but also help ease menstrual symptoms. So, here is a diet plan that will help you to not only manage weight loss and your symptoms but to gradually treat them both at the root.

- Morning drink- Ginger tea
- Breakfast- multigrain roti + 1 big bowl sabzi
- Mid-morning breakfast- apple with skin

- Lunch- 1 big bowl dal +1 small bowl curd
- Evening tea- kesar elaichi tea + 5 almonds (you can take 1 cube of 99% dark chocolate if you suffer from menstrual cramps)
- Dinner- 3-4 ragi idli with home made chutney
- Night drink- cinnamon tea + 1 small piece of gur

Benefits of these foods while being used in the diet for women wanting to manage menstrual symptoms while still working towards weight loss-:

- **Ginger:** Ginger has anti-inflammatory properties that can help alleviate menstrual cramps and reduce bloating. It may also aid in weight loss by boosting metabolism and reducing appetite.
- **Multigrains:** Whole grains like quinoa, brown rice, and whole wheat are rich in fiber, which can help regulate blood sugar levels and keep you feeling full, potentially aiding in weight management.
- **Sabzi (vegetables):** Vegetables provide essential nutrients and fiber, which can help with weight management and provide vitamins and minerals to support overall health.
- **Apple with skin:** Apples are a good source of fiber and can help regulate blood sugar levels and reduce cravings. The skin contains additional fiber and nutrients.
- **Dal (lentils):** Lentils are a great source of plant-based protein and fiber, which can help with weight loss and

provide long-lasting energy. They are also rich in iron, which can be beneficial during menstruation.

- **Curd (yogurt):** Yogurt provides probiotics that can aid in digestion and gut health. It's also a good source of protein and can help keep you full, supporting weight loss efforts.
- **Kesar (saffron) and Elaichi (cardamom):** These spices are often used in traditional remedies to alleviate menstrual discomfort. They can add flavor to dishes without added calories, making it easier to adhere to a weight loss plan.
- **Almonds:** Almonds are a source of healthy fats and protein, which can help with weight loss by promoting satiety. They also provide essential nutrients like magnesium and calcium.
- **Dark chocolate:** Dark chocolate in moderation can satisfy sweet cravings without consuming excessive calories. It may also improve mood, which can be beneficial during menstruation.
- **Ragi (finger millet):** Ragi is a whole grain rich in fiber and low in fat. It can help regulate blood sugar levels and support weight management.
- **Cinnamon tea:** Cinnamon has been associated with improved insulin sensitivity, which can help control blood sugar levels and reduce cravings. Drinking it as tea can be a low-calorie option.
- **Gur (jaggery):** Gur is a natural sweetener and is

considered a healthier alternative to refined sugar. It provides energy and can be used in moderation to satisfy sweet cravings.

Foods to Avoid or Limit during menstruation-:

- **Caffeine:** it can cause anxiety, irritability, breast tenderness and dehydration
- **Sugary Foods and Processed Snacks:** can lead to blood sugar spikes and crashes, which may worsen mood swings and cravings.
- **Salty Foods:** can cause water retention and bloating.
- **Dairy:** can exacerbate bloating and cramps.
- **Fatty and Fried Foods:** can increase inflammation and contribute to discomfort.
- **Alcohol:** Alcohol can worsen mood swings and may affect sleep quality.

2. Pregnancy-

We have discussed in the previous section about the process of menstruation. The formation of a mature egg in the ovaries every month, preparation and thickening of uterus lining and the descent of the egg into the uterus. The process after this is that the egg only lives here for 24 hours and if fertilization doesn't occur before the egg dies, it ends this process into menstruation. However, when the egg gets fertilized by the male sperm, this part of the process leads to pregnancy in the female body.

When someone is trying to conceive, this time frame of 24 hours is of utmost importance. And this is referred to as ovulation. Ovulation typically occurs approximately 14 days before the start of the next menstrual period, but the exact timing can vary among individuals and may not be the same in every menstrual cycle. Ovulation is the most fertile time in the menstrual cycle. Ovulation is regulated by a complex interplay of hormones, primarily luteinizing hormone (LH) and follicle-stimulating hormone (FSH). For some women predicting the occurrence of ovulation is easy as during this time they experience physical changes and few signs that signal the onset of ovulation. Other women use other methods to predict the onset of ovulation in order to conceive during this time.

You can predict ovulation using these common signs-

1. **Changes in Cervical Mucus:** it is another name for vaginal discharge. Nearing ovulation the cervical mucus becomes thinner, clearer(like raw egg white), stretchy and more slippery. Assess the texture of cervical mucus by taking it between your two fingers and you will notice that when you spread it, it forms long threads due to its increased thickness and stretchiness. This change in consistency and texture happens because it helps sperm travel through the cervix and into the uterus. To track the changes successfully you will have to start recording the consistency since the first day of your period cycle.
2. **Increased Libido:** Some individuals may experience an

increase in sexual desire and sensitivity around the time of ovulation. This happens to facilitate the possibility of sexual intercourse.

3. **Mild Pelvic Pain:** Some women experience a mild, dull ache on one side of the lower abdomen. Since we have two ovaries, each month the side of the ovary that releases the egg changes. One month, the left ovary releases the egg, the next month the right ovary. Pelvic pain occurs on the side from where the egg is released in that month. Not everyone feels this pain, and it can vary in intensity.
4. **Breast Tenderness:** Some women experience breast tenderness or soreness or tightness during ovulation, these symptoms are often caused by hormonal changes.
5. **Change in Basal Body Temperature:** To track the changes successfully you will have to keep record of your basal body temperature first thing in the morning before getting out of your bed, starting from the first day of your periods. Your BBT typically rises to one degree fahrenheit during ovulation due to the increase in progesterone.
6. **Mild Spotting:** In some cases, a small amount of spotting or vaginal bleeding can occur during ovulation. This is often referred to as ovulation bleeding.
7. **Positive Ovulation Test**: These test kits are like normal at-home pregnancy test kits. You have to put in a few drops of your urine into the test kit. It indicates a positive result by showing two pink lines. These tests are pretty

accurate, so you can use them as an additional factor for confirmation.

Unfortunately, for some couples, things do not always end up being easy as even after doing all the right things, they somehow fail to conceive a baby. There are many causes to the failure of conception which are not quite so apparent. If you and your partner have been trying for a period of 6 months now and all the efforts have proved to be futile, then there is a possibility that one of the following factors applies to you. However, I would always suggest you consult and confirm your conclusions with a doctor before finalizing them based on your personal views.

- **Irregular Menstrual Cycles:** Irregular or infrequent menstrual cycles can make it more challenging to pinpoint the fertile window, making conception less likely.
- **Absent ovulation/anovulation:** Conditions like polycystic ovary syndrome (PCOS), thyroid disorders, diabetes etc. can disrupt regular ovulation, reducing the chances of getting pregnant.
- **Stress:** High levels of stress can affect hormonal balance and may impact ovulation. It's essential to manage stress through relaxation techniques and lifestyle changes.
- **Uterine Issues OR fallopian blockage:** Endometriosis and in some cases the natural shape of the uterus can cause problems in implantation. Abnormalities in the uterus, such as fibroids or polyps, can also interfere with

implantation. Same ingrowths can cause fallopian tube blockage obstructing the pathway that connects ovaries to the uterus . When fallopian tubes are blocked, it can be hard for an egg and a sperm to meet. Additionally UTI, PID, SDI can also cause blockage of fallopian tubes.

- **Male Factors:** 20%-30% cases of infertility arise due to male factors. Issues like low sperm count, motility, or morphology can be factors causing fertilization or conception to fail. These can be detected using sperm analysis.
- **Age:** The age below 35 years for females and 40 years for males is considered the most fertile. Even when a female is in an ongoing menstrual cycle, after 35 years of age the quality of her egg gradually declines. Similarly, for males, the quality of sperm after 40 years of age, decreases as well. This factor can cause delay in fertilization and conception.
- **Weight:** Being underweight or overweight can affect fertility by disrupting hormonal balance.

Tips and tricks to successfully get pregnant-

1. Learn about your menstrual cycle & use ovulation kit- As I already stated above, after the egg descends towards the uterus, it stays alive only for 24 hours, however the sperm inside the female body can survive for 5-7 days. The best chances of fertilization are if the sperm remains there for a few days before, around and after

the egg descends from the ovaries. These days typically fall on the 12th, 13th, 14th, 15th and 16th days of a female's period cycle. Thus it is advisable to have sexual intercourse every second day starting from the 8th to 20th day of the period cycle.

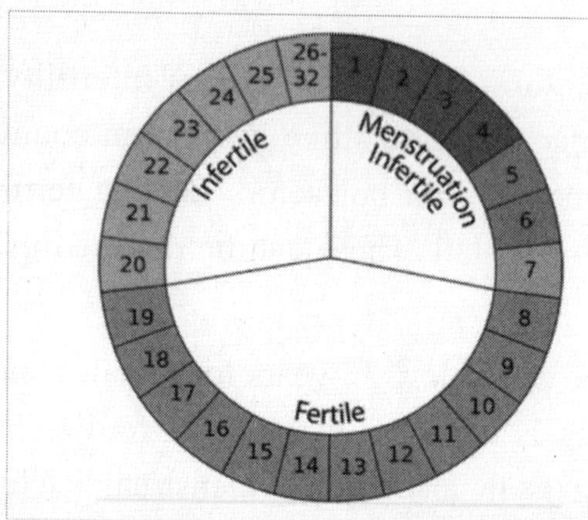

1. **Let go of birth control measures & vaginal lubricant-** It takes around 1 year for your body to return to normal hormonal levels after you stop taking birth control. So, let go of them as soon as you can. Also avoid using lubricants during intercourse as they can impede sperm movement.

2. **Weight-** You should keep optimum weight in order to conceive as being both overweight and underweight causes hindrances for pregnancy.

3. **Diet-** A diet rich in protein, vegetables, dry fruits, fruits & complex carbohydrates will aid in preparing the body for healthy pregnancy.

4. **Lifestyle changes-** Remember my 5 golden rules for a

healthy lifestyle, don't forget to include them here as well.

5. **Choose the right age-** As we discussed fertility is often considered high below the age of 35 years for women and below 40 for men.

6. **Multivitamin-**Start taking prenatal vitamins with folic acid and iron before conception. You should also include calcium supplements with these.

7. **No addiction-** Smoking, excessive alcohol and caffeine consumption reduces fertility. So, to conceive one should quit any kind of addiction that they have.

Even further if your problem still persists don't delay consultation with an expert doctor on the matter to get the help you need and deserve.

End note...

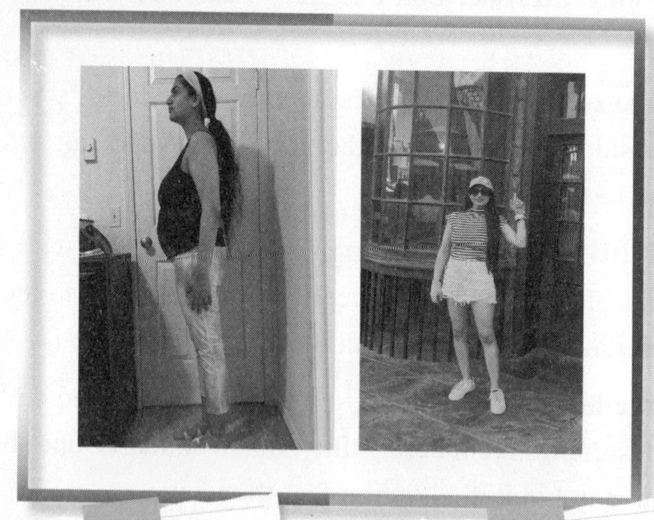

before

After

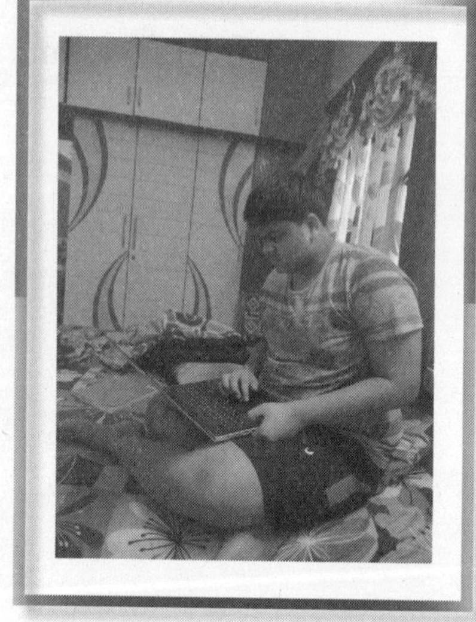

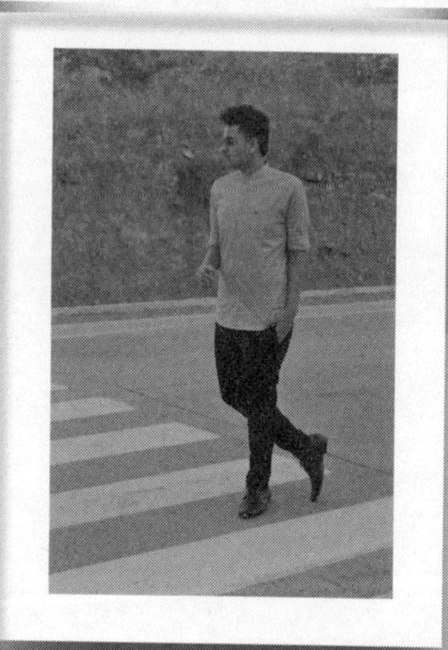

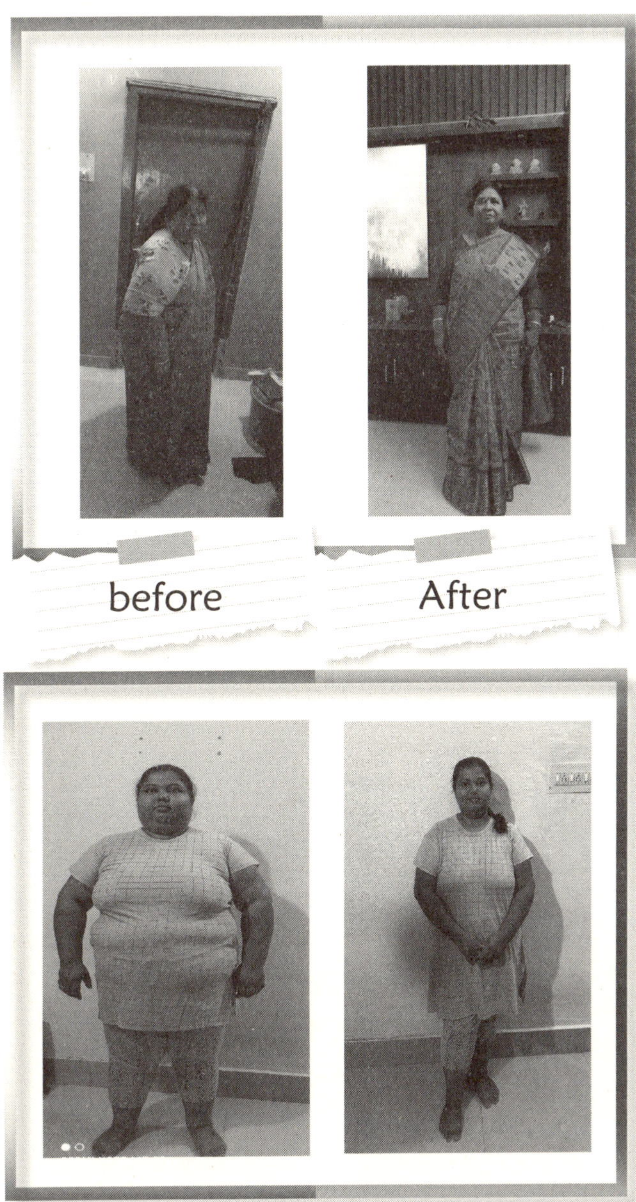
before
After

Note..